Future Research Needs Paper

Number 42

Treatment Strategies for Women With Coronary Artery Disease: Future Research Needs

Identification of Future Research Needs From Comparative Effectiveness Review No. 66

Prepared for:
Agency for Healthcare Research and Quality
U.S. Department of Health and Human Services
540 Gaither Road
Rockville, MD 20850
www.ahrq.gov

Contract No. 290-2007-10066-I

Prepared by:
Duke Evidence-based Practice Center
Durham, NC

Investigators:
Rowena J. Dolor, M.D., M.H.S.
Manesh R. Patel, M.D.
Chiara Melloni, M.D., M.H.S.
Ranee Chatterjee, M.D., M.P.H.
Brooke L. Heidenfelder, Ph.D.
Michael D. Musty, B.A.
Megan Chobot, M.S.L.S.
R. Julian Irvine, M.C.M.
Gillian D. Sanders, Ph.D

AHRQ Pub. No. 13-EHC073-EF
February 2013

This report is based on research conducted by the Duke Evidence-based Practice Center (EPC) under contract to the Agency for Healthcare Research and Quality (AHRQ), Rockville, MD (Contract No. 290-2007-10066-I). The findings and conclusions in this document are those of the author(s), who are responsible for its contents; the findings and conclusions do not necessarily represent the views of AHRQ. Therefore, no statement in this report should be construed as an official position of AHRQ or of the U.S. Department of Health and Human Services.

The information in this report is intended to help health care researchers and funders of research make well-informed decisions in designing and funding research and thereby improve the quality of health care services. This report is not intended to be a substitute for the application of scientific judgment. Anyone who makes decisions concerning the provision of clinical care should consider this report in the same way as any medical research and in conjunction with all other pertinent information, i.e., in the context of available resources and circumstances.

This document is in the public domain and may be used and reprinted without permission except those copyrighted materials that are clearly noted in the document. Further reproduction of those copyrighted materials is prohibited without the specific permission of copyright holders.

Persons using assistive technology may not be able to fully access information in this report. For assistance contact EffectiveHealthCare@ahrq.hhs.gov.

Suggested citation: Dolor, RJ, Patel MR, Melloni C, Chatterjee R, Heidenfelder BL, Musty MD, Chobot M, Irvine RJ, Sanders GD. Treatment Strategies for Women With Coronary Artery Disease: Future Research Needs. Future Research Needs Paper No. 42. (Prepared by the Duke Evidence-based Practice Center under Contract No. 290-2007-10066-I). AHRQ Publication No. 13-EHC073-EF. Rockville, MD: Agency for Healthcare Research and Quality. February 2013. www.effectivehealthcare.ahrq.gov/reports.final.cfm.

Preface

The Agency for Healthcare Research and Quality (AHRQ), through its Evidence-based Practice Centers (EPCs), sponsors the development of evidence reports and technology assessments to assist public- and private-sector organizations in their efforts to improve the quality of health care in the United States. The reports and assessments provide organizations with comprehensive, science-based information on common, costly medical conditions and new health care technologies and strategies. The EPCs systematically review the relevant scientific literature on topics assigned to them by AHRQ and conduct additional analyses when appropriate prior to developing their reports and assessments.

An important part of evidence reports is to not only synthesize the evidence, but also to identify the gaps in evidence that limited the ability to answer the systematic review questions. AHRQ supports EPCs to work with various stakeholders to identify and prioritize the future research that are needed by decisionmakers. This information is provided for researchers and funders of research in these Future Research Needs papers. These papers are made available for public comment and use and may be revised.

AHRQ expects that the EPC evidence reports and technology assessments will inform individual health plans, providers, and purchasers as well as the health care system as a whole by providing important information to help improve health care quality. The evidence reports undergo public comment prior to their release as a final report.

We welcome comments on this Future Research Needs document. They may be sent by mail to the Task Order Officer named below at: Agency for Healthcare Research and Quality, 540 Gaither Road, Rockville, MD 20850, or by email to epc@ahrq.hhs.gov.

Carolyn M. Clancy, M.D.
Director
Agency for Healthcare Research and Quality

Jean Slutsky, P.A., M.S.P.H.
Director, Center for Outcomes and Evidence
Agency for Healthcare Research and Quality

Stephanie Chang M.D., M.P.H.
Director, EPC Program
Center for Outcomes and Evidence
Agency for Healthcare Research and Quality

Elisabeth Kato, M.D.
Task Order Officer
Center for Outcomes and Evidence
Agency for Healthcare Research and Quality

Acknowledgments

The authors thank Megan von Isenburg, M.L.S., for help with the literature search and retrieval, and Elizabeth Wing, M.A., for editorial assistance.

Stakeholders

Lisa Begg, Dr.P.H., R.N.
Director of Research Programs
National Institutes of Health
Office of Research on Women's Health
Bethesda, MD

Peter Berger, M.D., FACC, FAHA, FSCAI
Vice-Chairman, Cardiology
Director, Center for Clinical Studies
Geisinger Health System
Danville, PA

Brenda J. Clark
Patient Advocate
Go Red for Women
American Heart Association
San Francisco, CA

Nakela L. Cook, M.D., M.P.H.
Clinical Medical Officer
National Heart, Lung and Blood Institute
Bethesda, MD

Bernice Hecker, M.D., M.H.A., FACC
Medical Director, Noridian Administrative
Services (Medicare contractor)
Fargo, ND

Linda Humphrey, M.D., M.P.H.
Clinical Director
Evidence-based Synthesis Program
Portland Veterans Affairs Medical Center
Portland, OR

Eugenie Komives, M.D.
Former Vice President and Sr. Medical
  Director
Blue Cross Blue Shield of North Carolina
Durham, NC

Lori Mosca, M.D., Ph.D., M.P.H.
Professor of Medicine
Director of Preventive Cardiology
Columbia University Medical Center
New York–Presbyterian Hospital
New York, NY

John Puskas, M.D., M.Sc.
Professor of Surgery and Associate Chief
Division of Cardiothoracic Surgery
Emory University School of Medicine
Chief of Cardiac Surgery
Emory University Hospital-Midtown
Atlanta, GA

Kimberly Skelding, M.D.
Director, Cardiovascular Genomics and
  Cardiovascular Research
Geisinger Health System
Danville, PA

Contents

Executive Summary

Background

Cardiovascular disease remains the leading cause of death among women in the United States.[1] More than 500,000 women die of cardiovascular disease each year, exceeding the number of deaths in men and the next seven causes of death in women combined. This translates into approximately one death every minute.[1,2] This report focuses on women because of the differences in clinical presentation and extent and location of coronary disease on presentation, which affect the treatment options for coronary artery disease (CAD).[3-5] Currently available guidelines and systematic reviews provide specific treatment recommendations for women only among a subset of treatment options, and overall assume that treatment options are equally effective for both sexes when gender data are not available. However, women have a worse prognosis than men for manifestations of CAD such as acute myocardial infarction, and some data suggest that women and men may not respond equally to the same treatments. Further, women are more likely than men to experience bleeding complications.[6-9]

In 2012, a Comparative Effectiveness Review (CER), "Treatment Strategies for Women With Coronary Artery Disease," attempted to assess the comparative effectiveness of the major treatment options for CAD specifically in women, evaluating these comparisons[10]:

1. Percutaneous coronary intervention (PCI) versus fibrinolysis or PCI versus conservative/supportive medical management in women with ST elevation myocardial infarction (STEMI)
2. Early invasive versus initial conservative management in women with unstable angina or non-ST elevation myocardial infarction (UA/NSTEMI)
3. PCI versus coronary artery bypass graft surgery (CABG) versus optimal medical therapy in women with stable or unstable angina

Twenty-eight comparative studies contributed evidence about effectiveness, modifiers of effectiveness, or safety for the comparisons above. For women with STEMI, five studies showed a reduction in composite outcomes (primarily death/myocardial infarction (MI)/stroke) at 30 days for PCI over fibrinolysis (odds ratio [OR] 0.50; 95% confidence interval [CI], 0.36 to 0.72; high strength of evidence [SOE]); there was insufficient evidence for assessing outcomes at 1 year. For women with UA/NSTEMI, the included studies, although not showing statistical significance, suggested a benefit of early invasive over initial conservative management for the composite outcome of primarily death/MI at 6 months and (2 studies OR 0.77; 95% CI, 0.28 to 2.12; low SOE; 5 studies OR 0.78; 95% CI, 0.54 to 1.12; low SOE). Evidence suggested a small benefit of initial conservative management at 5 years (2 studies, OR 1.05; 95% CI, 0.81 to 1.35; insufficient SOE); however, with the wide confidence interval crossing 1, and the trend favoring early invasive therapy suggested at earlier time points, we cannot support firm conclusions. For women with stable angina randomized to revascularization (PCI or CABG) or medical therapy, four studies showed a reduction in the composite outcome of death/MI/repeat revascularization at 5 years for revascularization with either PCI (OR 0.64; 95% CI, 0.47 to 0.89; moderate SOE) or CABG (OR 0.56; 95% CI, 0.32 to 0.96; low SOE). For stable and unstable angina trials comparing PCI with CABG, two studies suggested a nonsignificant benefit of PCI in reducing mortality at 30 days (low SOE). At 1 year and beyond, although suggestive of a benefit of CABG for the composite outcomes of death/MI/stroke for women, this finding was not statistically significant and represented wide confidence intervals (low SOE at 1 year and at >2 years).

Five studies assessed modifiers of effectiveness in women due to demographic factors (≥65 or ≥80 years of age) or clinical factors (risk stratification or diabetes). Strength of evidence for modifiers of effectiveness for STEMI, NSTEMI, and stable/unstable angina was insufficient.

Four studies assessed safety outcomes in women: two STEMI studies (PCI vs. fibrinolysis) and two NSTEMI studies (PCI vs. CABG) assessed transfusion rates, incidence of intracranial hemorrhage, and bleeding rates. Strength of evidence for safety outcomes for all the CAD presentations was insufficient.

Given the clinical and economic importance of treating CAD in women, the ongoing investment in CAD research on medical therapy, PCI and CABG, and the remaining areas of uncertainty, we sought to create a prioritized future research agenda that would represent the interests of diverse stakeholders and allow the remaining areas of uncertainty to be addressed.

Analytic Framework

A number of areas for future research were identified in the CER. We have organized these evidence gaps according to the patient, intervention/comparator, and outcomes (PICO) format. We have categorized these areas for potential future research in the table below (Table A), and mapped them into the Analytic Framework presented in Figure A.

Table A. Initial list of evidence gaps

PICO Element	Evidence Gaps
Population	1. Is there evidence that the comparative effectiveness of PCI vs. fibrinolysis/supportive therapy in women with STEMI; early invasive vs. initial conservative therapy in women with UA/NSTEMI; or PCI vs. CABG or revascularization vs. optimal medical therapy in women with stable or unstable angina differs by such characteristics as: a. **Age, race, or other demographic and socioeconomic risk factors?** b. **Coronary disease risk factors** such as diabetes, chronic kidney disease, or other comorbid disease? c. **Angiographic-specific factors** (number of diseased vessels, vessel territory stenoses, left ventricular function, access site, or prior PCI or CABG revascularization procedure)? d. **Hospital characteristics** (hospital volume, setting, guideline-based treatment protocols)?

Table A. Initial list of evidence gaps (continued)

PICO Element	Evidence Gaps

Intervention and Comparator	2. In women presenting with *STEMI*: What is the effectiveness of PCI vs. fibrinolysis/supportive therapy **on intermediate- or long-term** clinical outcomes (nonfatal MI, death, stroke, repeat revascularization, recurrent unstable angina, heart failure, repeat hospitalization, length of hospital stay, angina relief, quality of life, or cognitive effects)?
	3. In women presenting with *UA/NSTEMI*: What is the effectiveness of early invasive (PCI or CABG) vs. initial conservative therapy **on short-, intermediate- or long-term** clinical outcomes (nonfatal MI, death, stroke, repeat revascularization, recurrent unstable angina, heart failure, repeat hospitalization, length of hospital stay, graft failure, angina relief, quality of life, or cognitive effects)?
	4. In women presenting with *stable or unstable angina*: What is the effectiveness of the following treatment strategies on **short-, intermediate- or long-term** clinical outcomes (nonfatal MI, death, stroke, repeat revascularization, recurrent unstable angina, heart failure, repeat hospitalization, length of hospital stay, graft failure, angina relief, quality of life, or cognitive effects)?
	   a. Revascularization (PCI or CABG) vs. optimal medical therapy in women with stable angina
	   b. PCI vs. CABG in women with stable or unstable angina

Outcome	5. What are the **potential harms** in women of:
	   a. PCI vs. fibrinolysis/supportive therapy with STEMI?
	   b. Early invasive vs. initial conservative therapy with UA/NSTEMI?
	   c. PCI vs. CABG or revascularization vs. optimal medical therapy with stable or unstable angina?

Abbreviations: CABG = coronary artery bypass graft surgery; MI = myocardial infarction; PCI = percutaneous coronary intervention; STEMI = ST elevation myocardial infarction; UA/NSTEMI = unstable angina/non-ST elevation myocardial infarction

ES-3

Figure A. Analytic framework

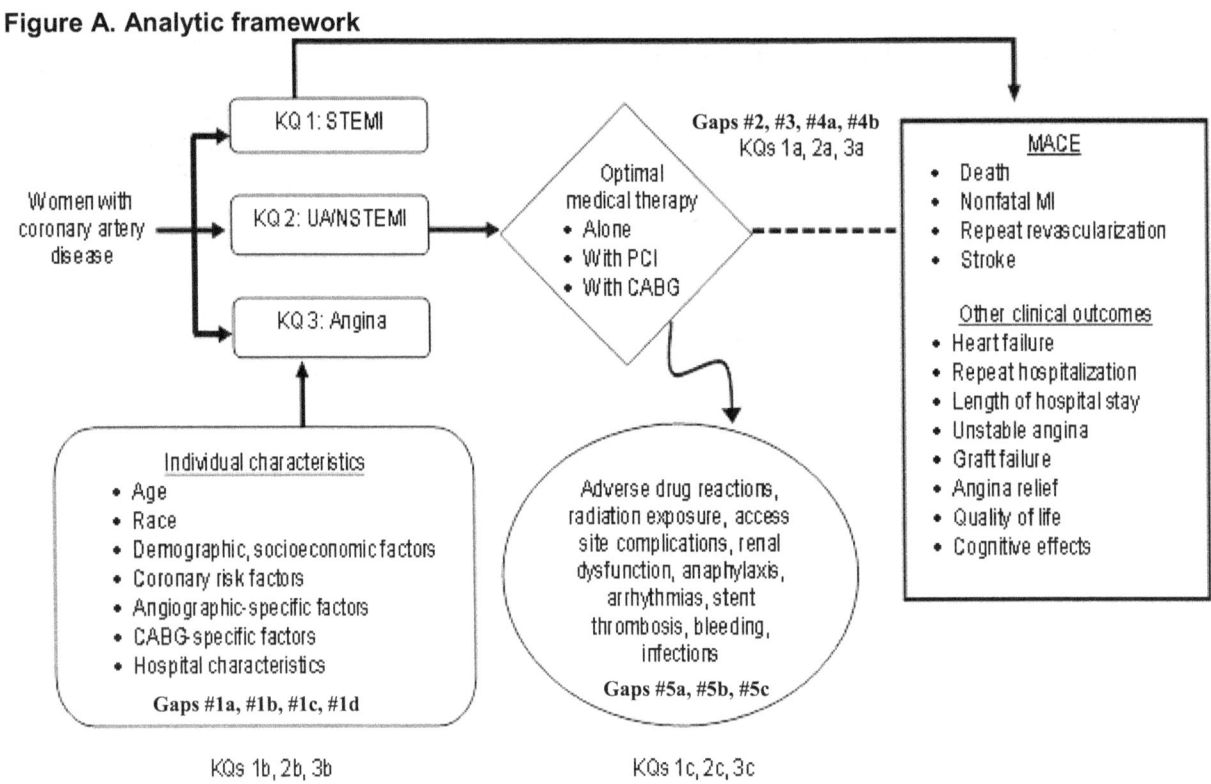

Abbreviations: CABG = coronary artery bypass graft; KQ = Key Question; MACE = major adverse cardiovascular events; MI = myocardial infarction; NSTEMI = non-ST elevation myocardial infarction; PCI = percutaneous coronary intervention; STEMI = ST elevation myocardial infarction; UA/NSTEMI = unstable angina/non-ST elevation myocardial infarction.

Methods

Our approach to identifying evidence gaps, prioritizing future research, and developing recommendations for stakeholders is outlined in the following steps.

1. Develop an analytic framework from the original CER in order to understand the clinical and policy context of the review and its initial list of Future Research Needs.
2. Create an initial list of evidence gaps based on the CER organized according to the PICOframework.[11]
3. Form a stakeholder group representing appropriate clinician, policymaker, and patient perspectives.
4. Expand the list of evidence gaps based on stakeholder input.
5. Perform an updated review of published literature since the last CER (search last updated in December 2011) and a horizon scan for recently published and ongoing studies that may address the evidence gaps, but which are not included in the current CER.
6. Solicit stakeholder prioritization of the identified research gaps based on the updated literature review.
7. Determine the most appropriate study designs for the highest priority research areas.[12]

Stakeholders were selected to include a broad range of stakeholder perspectives, including researchers involved in some of the primary randomized controlled trials (RCTs) included in the CER, other clinical experts and researchers in the content area, representatives from Federal and nongovernmental funding agencies, representatives from relevant professional societies, health care decision- and policymakers, and representatives from related consumer and patient advocacy groups. We started with the main research priorities identified in the original CER, and breaking out each sub-section into its own evidence gap resulted in a list of 13 research priorities, including implementation gaps. Based on input from the stakeholder workgroup during the first call, we ultimately expanded the list of research priorities to a total of 15. After the second stakeholder call, it was decided that one of the research priorities needed to be removed since it essentially encompassed all of the other research priorities, thus leaving 14 for the second ranking.

We performed three database searches to identify ongoing and recently published studies relevant to the identified evidence gaps. These included a search of ClinicalTrials.gov, an update of the PubMed, Embase, and Cochrane searches used in the original CER, and a search of PubMed® for relevant systematic reviews that may address the evidence gaps considered out of scope in the original review. Based on these searches, a document was created listing all included articles and clinical trials that might pertain to the initial 15 listed evidence gaps.

The stakeholders were provided with the AHRQ Effective Health Care Program prioritization criteria for Future Research Needs and instructed to use these criteria as the basis for their decisions regarding research prioritization. The stakeholders performed two online rankings of the identified research priorities (including the additional priorities identified by the stakeholder team). This ranking utilized a forced-ranking prioritization method, whereby participants were given 5 votes to allocate to any of the 14–15 research priorities, with a maximum of 3 votes per item.

For the top tier Future Research Needs, we considered potential study designs and their advantages and disadvantages.[12] While these proposed methods to address each area are not intended to be restrictive of potential study designs, we comment on each design's potential benefits or limitations for answering these questions.

Results

Based on the 2012 CER, "Treatment Strategies for Women With Coronary Artery Disease,"[10] and our discussion with stakeholders, we initially identified 15 potential research areas, which were then reduced to 14 areas. The stakeholder voting identified two highest priority areas of future research in each prioritization exercise. The highest priority area from the first prioritization was removed after discussion with the stakeholders, as it was comprehensive of the other research areas and was potentially skewing the rest of the rankings. After the second prioritization, there was just one highest priority area: the second-highest ranked gap from the first prioritization. Initially it was only separated from next-highest ranked gap by 2 points, but after the second prioritization exercise, this separation increased to 8 points and therefore was listed as the sole high priority research area. The results were somewhat different between the two separate prioritization exercises for the middle and lower tiers, as was expected with the removal of the overarching research area; however there was still no great separation between the middle and lower tiers. The research priorities are shown in Table B.

Table B. Final ranking of Future Research Needs for treatment strategies for women with CAD

Tier	Question	Score
Top Tier	What is the effectiveness of the following treatment strategies on short-, intermediate- or long-term clinical outcomes (nonfatal MI, death, stroke, repeat revascularization, recurrent unstable angina, heart failure, repeat hospitalization, length of hospital stay, graft failure, angina relief, quality of life, or cognitive effects)? **Revascularization (PCI or CABG) vs. optimal medical therapy in women with unstable angina**	13
Middle Tier	Is there evidence that the comparative effectiveness of PCI vs. fibrinolysis/supportive therapy in women with STEMI; early invasive vs. initial conservative therapy in women with UA/NSTEMI; or PCI vs. CABG or revascularization vs. optimal medical therapy in women with stable or unstable angina differs by such characteristics as: **Coronary disease risk factors such as diabetes, chronic kidney disease, or other comorbid disease?**	5
	What is the effectiveness of the following treatment strategies on short-, intermediate- or long-term clinical outcomes (nonfatal MI, death, stroke, repeat revascularization, recurrent unstable angina, heart failure, repeat hospitalization, length of hospital stay, graft failure, angina relief, quality of life, or cognitive effects)? **PCI vs. CABG in women with stable or unstable angina**	4
	What are the potential harms in women of PCI vs. CABG or revascularization vs. optimal medical therapy with stable or unstable angina?	4
	*Are the **patient outcomes from real-world settings** or observational registries similar to the findings from randomized clinical trials?**	4
	Is there evidence that the comparative effectiveness of PCI vs. fibrinolysis/supportive therapy in women with STEMI; early invasive vs. initial conservative therapy in women with UA/NSTEMI; or PCI vs. CABG or revascularization vs. optimal medical therapy in women with stable or unstable angina differs by such characteristics as: **Angiographic-specific factors (number of diseased vessels, vessel territory stenoses, left ventricular function, access site, or prior PCI or CABG revascularization procedure)?**	3
	*Does **patient preference or clinical specialty** (primary care, cardiology, cardiothoracic surgery) affect the choice of treatment strategy (medical therapy or type of revascularization)?**	3
Lower Tier	Is there evidence that the comparative effectiveness of PCI vs. fibrinolysis/supportive therapy in women with STEMI; early invasive vs. initial conservative therapy in women with UA/NSTEMI; or PCI vs. CABG or revascularization vs. optimal medical therapy in women with stable or unstable angina differs by such characteristics as: **Age, race, or other demographic and socioeconomic risk factors?**	2
	In women presenting with STEMI: What is the effectiveness of **PCI vs. fibrinolysis/supportive therapy** on intermediate- or long-term clinical outcomes (nonfatal MI, death, stroke, repeat revascularization, recurrent unstable angina, heart failure, repeat hospitalization, length of hospital stay, angina relief, quality of life, or cognitive effects)?	2
	In women presenting with UA/NSTEMI: What is the effectiveness of **early invasive (PCI or CABG) vs. initial conservative therapy** on short-, intermediate- or long-term clinical outcomes (nonfatal MI, death, stroke, repeat revascularization, recurrent unstable angina, heart failure, repeat hospitalization, length of hospital stay, graft failure, angina relief, quality of life, or cognitive effects)?	2
	*Are there **gender differences** in the instruments used to measure functional status, risk factors, comorbidities, etc. associated with CAD?**	2
	What are the **potential harms** in women of early invasive vs. initial conservative therapy with UA/NSTEMI?	2
	Is there evidence that the comparative effectiveness of PCI vs. fibrinolysis/supportive therapy in women with STEMI; early invasive vs. initial conservative therapy in women with UA/NSTEMI; or PCI vs. CABG or revascularization vs. optimal medical therapy in women with stable or unstable angina differs by such characteristics as: **Hospital characteristics** (hospital volume, setting, guideline-based treatment protocols)?	1
	What are the **potential harms** in women of PCI vs. fibrinolysis/supportive therapy with STEMI?	1

Abbreviations: CABG = coronary artery bypass graft surgery; CAD = coronary artery disease; MI = myocardial infarction; PCI = percutaneous coronary intervention; STEMI = ST elevation myocardial infarction; UA/NSTEMI = unstable angina/non-ST elevation myocardial infarction
*Out-of-scope research topics are highlighted in italics.

Discussion

The recommendations for future research prioritization of treatment strategies in this report represents the perspectives of a broad range of stakeholders, including researchers involved in some of the primary RCTs included in the CER, other clinical experts and researchers in the content area, representatives from Federal and nongovernmental funding agencies, representatives from relevant professional societies, health care decisionmakers and policymakers, and representatives from related consumer and patient advocacy groups. The top tier of two research priorities differed slightly between our first and second prioritization exercise due to the removal of one research area. The two areas in the final ranking represent two primary foci: (1) clinical decisionmaking (i.e., the effect of treatment decisions on clinical outcomes); and (2) implementation and generalizability (i.e., the effect of risk factors and comorbid disease on treatment outcomes).

The stakeholder group included a few topics that were out of the scope of the original review, but which are related to issues occurring in actual practice. While the original search strategy may have identified studies addressing these topics, these outcomes were not part of the outcomes of interest in the CER and so there is no available summary of the strength of evidence. The expansion of topics promotes consideration of new areas of research that have not been adequately explored, and this is evidenced by the literature scan in this report, which was unable to identify any articles of relevance to these out-of-scope topics. Nevertheless, the original CER did not comment on the state of current research in these out-of-scope areas, and they should only be promoted with the caveat that the existing literature may already adequately address these areas.

Conclusions

A workgroup of 10 stakeholders identified the following research area as the highest priority for future research for the comparative effectiveness of treatment strategies for women with CAD.

1. In women presenting with stable or unstable angina: What is the effectiveness of the following treatment strategies on short-, intermediate- or long-term clinical outcomes (i.e., nonfatal MI, death, stroke, repeat revascularization, recurrent unstable angina, heart failure, repeat hospitalization, length of hospital stay, graft failure, angina relief, quality of life, or cognitive effects)? **Revascularization (PCI or CABG) versus optimal medical therapy in women with unstable angina**
   a. Recommended study design: (preferable) large long-term clinical trial with women-only enrollment or of large enough sample size with stratification of randomization by sex to allow for meaningful sex-based analyses; also possible would be meta-analyses of all existing clinical trials with patient-level data to more accurately describe sex-stratified outcomes

References

1. Roger VL, Go AS, Lloyd-Jones DM, et al. Heart Disease and Stroke Statistics--2012 update: a report from the American Heart Association. Circulation. 2012 Jan 3;125(1):e2-e220. PMID: 22179539.

2. Mosca L, Banka CL, Benjamin EJ, et al. Evidence-based guidelines for cardiovascular disease prevention in women: 2007 update. Circulation. 2007 Mar 20;115(11):1481-501. PMID: 17309915.

3. Shaw LJ, Bugiardini R, Merz CN. Women and ischemic heart disease: evolving knowledge. J Am Coll Cardiol. 2009 Oct 20;54(17):1561-75. PMID: 19833255.

4. Hochman JS, Tamis JE, Thompson TD, et al. Sex, clinical presentation, and outcome in patients with acute coronary syndromes. Global Use of Strategies to Open Occluded Coronary Arteries in Acute Coronary Syndromes IIb Investigators. N Engl J Med. 1999 July 22;341(4):226-32. PMID: 10413734.

5. Berger JS, Elliott L, Gallup D, et al. Sex differences in mortality following acute coronary syndromes. JAMA. 2009 Aug 26;302(8):874-82. PMID: 19706861.

6. Mieres JH, Shaw LJ, Arai A, et al. Role of noninvasive testing in the clinical evaluation of women with suspected coronary artery disease: consensus statement from the Cardiac Imaging Committee, Council on Clinical Cardiology, and the Cardiovascular Imaging and Intervention Committee, Council on Cardiovascular Radiology and Intervention, American Heart Association. Circulation. 2005 Feb 8;111(5):682-96. PMID: 15687114.

7. Alexander KP, Chen AY, Newby LK, et al. Sex differences in major bleeding with glycoprotein IIb/IIIa inhibitors: results from the CRUSADE (Can Rapid risk stratification of Unstable angina patients Suppress ADverse outcomes with Early implementation of the ACC/AHA guidelines) initiative. Circulation. 2006 Sep 26;114(13):1380-7. PMID: 16982940.

8. Pepine CJ. Ischemic heart disease in women: facts and wishful thinking. J Am Coll Cardiol. 2004 May 19;43(10):1727-30. PMID: 15145090.

9. Vaccarino V, Abramson JL, Veledar E, et al. Sex differences in hospital mortality after coronary artery bypass surgery: evidence for a higher mortality in younger women. Circulation. 2002 Mar 12;105(10):1176-81. PMID: 11889010.

10. Dolor RJ, Melloni C, Chatterjee R, et al. Treatment Strategies for Women With Coronary Artery Disease. Comparative Effectiveness Review No. 66. (Prepared by the Duke Evidence-based Practice Center under Contract No. 290-2007-10066-I.) AHRQ Publication No. 12-EHC070-EF. Rockville, MD: Agency for Healthcare Research and Quality. August 2012. www.effectivehealthcare.ahrq.gov/reports/final.cfm.

11. Robinson KA, Saldanha IJ, McKoy NA. Development of a framework to identify research gaps from systematic reviews. J Clin Epidemiol. 2011 Dec;64(12):1325-30. PMID: 21937195.

12. Carey T, Sanders GD, Viswanathan M, et al. Framework for Considering Study Designs for Future Research Needs. Methods Future Research Needs Paper No. 8. (Prepared by the RTI–UNC Evidence-based Practice Center under Contract No. 290-2007-10056-I.) AHRQ Publication No. 12-EHC048-EF. Rockville, MD: Agency for Healthcare Research and Quality. March 2012. www.effectivehealthcare.ahrq.gov/reports/final.cfm.

Background

Cardiovascular disease remains the leading cause of death among women in the United States.[1] More than 500,000 women die of cardiovascular disease each year, exceeding the number of deaths in men and the next seven causes of death in women combined. This translates into approximately one death every minute.[1,2] This report focuses on women because of the differences in clinical presentation and coronary anatomy, which affect the treatment options for coronary artery disease (CAD).[3-5] Currently available guidelines and systematic reviews provide specific treatment recommendations for women only among a subset of treatment options, and overall assume that treatment options are equally effective for both sexes when gender data are not available. However, women have a worse prognosis than men for manifestations of CAD such as acute myocardial infarction (MI), and some data suggest that women and men do not respond equally to the same treatments. Further, women are more likely than men to experience bleeding complications.[6-9]

In 2012, a Comparative Effectiveness Review (CER), "Treatment Strategies for Women With Coronary Artery Disease," attempted to assess the comparative effectiveness of the major treatment options for CAD specifically in women, evaluating these comparisons[10]:

1. Percutaneous coronary intervention (PCI) versus fibrinolysis or PCI versus conservative/supportive medical management in women with ST elevation myocardial infarction (STEMI)
2. Early invasive versus initial conservative management in women with unstable angina or non-ST elevation myocardial infarction (UA/NSTEMI)
3. PCI versus coronary artery bypass graft surgery (CABG) versus optimal medical therapy in women with stable or unstable angina

The CER addressed the following three Key Questions (KQs):

- **KQ 1.** In women presenting with STEMI:
  a. What is the effectiveness of PCI versus fibrinolysis/supportive therapy on clinical outcomes (e.g., nonfatal MI, death, stroke, repeat revascularization, recurrent unstable angina, heart failure, repeat hospitalization, length of hospital stay, angina relief, quality of life, or cognitive effects)?
  b. Is there evidence that the comparative effectiveness of PCI versus fibrinolysis/supportive therapy varies based on characteristics such as:
     - Age, race, or other demographic and socioeconomic risk factors?
     - Coronary disease risk factors such as diabetes, chronic kidney disease, or other comorbid disease?
     - Angiographic-specific factors (i.e., number of diseased vessels, vessel territory stenoses, left ventricular function, access site, or prior PCI or CABG revascularization procedure)?
     - Hospital characteristics (e.g., hospital volume, setting, guideline-based treatment protocols)?
  c. What are the significant safety concerns associated with each treatment strategy (e.g., adverse drug reactions, radiation exposure, access site complications, renal dysfunction, anaphylaxis, arrhythmias, stent thrombosis, bleeding, infections)?

- **KQ 2.** In women presenting with UA/NSTEMI:
  a. What is the effectiveness of early invasive (PCI or CABG) versus initial conservative therapy on clinical outcomes (e.g., nonfatal MI, death, stroke, repeat revascularization, recurrent unstable angina, heart failure, repeat hospitalization, length of hospital stay, graft failure, angina relief, quality of life, or cognitive effects)?
  b. Is there evidence that the comparative effectiveness of early invasive versus initial conservative therapy varies based on characteristics such as:
     – Age, race, or other demographic and socioeconomic risk factors?
     – Coronary disease risk factors such as diabetes, chronic kidney disease, or other comorbid disease?
     – Angiographic-specific factors (i.e., number of diseased vessels, vessel territory stenoses, left ventricular function, access site, or prior PCI or CABG revascularization procedure)?
     – Hospital characteristics (e.g., hospital volume, setting, guideline-based treatment protocols)?
  c. What are the significant safety concerns associated with each treatment strategy (e.g., adverse drug reactions, radiation exposure, access site complications, renal dysfunction, anaphylaxis, arrhythmias, stent thrombosis, bleeding, infections)?
- **KQ 3.** In women presenting with stable or unstable angina:
  a. What is the effectiveness of the following treatment strategies on clinical outcomes (e.g., nonfatal MI, death, stroke, repeat revascularization, recurrent unstable angina, heart failure, repeat hospitalization, length of hospital stay, graft failure, angina relief, quality of life, or cognitive effects)?
     – Revascularization (PCI or CABG) versus optimal medical therapy in women with stable angina
     – PCI versus CABG in women with stable or unstable angina
  b. Is there evidence that the comparative effectiveness of revascularization versus optimal medical therapy varies based on characteristics such as:
     – Age, race, or other demographic and socioeconomic risk factors?
     – Coronary disease risk factors such as diabetes, chronic kidney disease, or other comorbid disease?
     – Angiographic-specific factors (i.e., number of diseased vessels, vessel territory stenoses, left ventricular function, access site, or prior PCI or CABG revascularization procedure)?
     – CABG-specific factors such as type of surgery performed, cardiopulmonary bypass mode (normothermic versus hypothermic), on-pump versus off-pump, type of cardioplegia used (blood versus crystalloid), or use of saphenous vein grafts, single or bilateral internal mammary artery grafts, or other types of bypass grafts
     – Hospital characteristics (e.g., hospital volume, setting, guideline-based treatment protocols)?
  c. What are the significant safety concerns associated with each treatment strategy (e.g., adverse drug reactions, radiation exposure, access site

2

complications, renal dysfunction, anaphylaxis, arrhythmias, stent thrombosis, bleeding, infections)?

Twenty-eight comparative studies contributed evidence about effectiveness, modifiers of effectiveness, or safety for the comparisons above. For women with STEMI, five studies showed a reduction in composite outcomes (primarily death/MI/stroke) at 30 days for PCI over fibrinolysis (odds ratio [OR] 0.50; 95% confidence interval [CI], 0.36 to 0.72; high strength of evidence [SOE]); there was insufficient evidence for assessing outcomes at 1 year. For women with UA/NSTEMI, the included studies, although not showing statistical significance, suggested a benefit of early invasive over initial conservative management for the composite outcome of primarily death/MI at 6 months and (2 studies OR 0.77; 95% CI, 0.28 to 2.12; low SOE; 5 studies OR 0.78; 95% CI, 0.54 to 1.12; low SOE). Evidence suggested a small benefit of initial conservative management at 5 years (2 studies, OR 1.05; 95% CI, 0.81 to 1.35; insufficient SOE); however, with the wide confidence interval crossing 1, and the trend favoring early invasive therapy suggested at earlier time points, we cannot support firm conclusions. For women with stable angina randomized to revascularization (PCI or CABG) or medical therapy, four studies showed a reduction in the composite outcome of death/MI/repeat revascularization at 5 years for revascularization with either PCI (OR 0.64; 95% CI, 0.47 to 0.89; moderate SOE) or CABG (OR 0.56; 95% CI, 0.32 to 0.96; low SOE). For stable and unstable angina trials comparing PCI with CABG, two studies suggested a nonsignificant benefit of PCI in reducing mortality at 30 days (low SOE). At 1 year and beyond, although suggestive of a benefit of CABG for the composite outcomes of death/MI/stroke for women, this finding was not statistically significant and represented wide confidence intervals (low SOE at 1 year and at >2 years).

Five studies assessed modifiers of effectiveness in women due to demographic factors (≥65 or ≥80 years of age) or clinical factors (risk stratification or diabetes). Strength of evidence for modifiers of effectiveness for STEMI, NSTEMI, and stable/unstable angina was insufficient. Four studies assessed safety outcomes in women: two STEMI studies (PCI vs. fibrinolysis) and two NSTEMI studies (PCI vs. CABG) assessed transfusion rates, incidence of intracranial hemorrhage, and bleeding rates. Strength of evidence for safety outcomes for all the CAD presentations was insufficient.

The weaknesses and shortcomings of the evidence base identified during the review confirmed that more research is needed. Therefore, this Future Research Needs prioritization seeks to review and identify the evidence gaps in the treatment strategies for women with coronary artery disease, and to prioritize the focus and design of future research comparing these modalities. Summary of the evidence and key findings from the review are shown in Table 1.

3

Table 1. Summary of key findings

Key Question	Strength of Evidence	Conclusions
KQ 1: Women with STEMI (PCI vs. fibrinolysis/supportive therapy)	Effectiveness of intervention 1. High (women and men) for short-term (30-day) composite outcomes 2. Insufficient (women and men) for intermediate-term (1-year) composite outcomes Modifiers of effectiveness Insufficient Safety concerns Insufficient	7 studies (6 good quality, 1 fair) compared PCI with or without supportive therapy to fibrinolysis or other routine medical care for women with STEMI and contributed evidence about the comparative effectiveness, modifiers of effectiveness, or safety for these interventions. These studies included a total of 4527 patients, of which 1174 (26%) were women. • Effectiveness of interventions: A meta-analysis of 5 studies (all good quality) reporting 30-day composite outcomes (primarily death/MI/stroke) showed that PCI was better than fibrinolysis in women (OR, 0.50; 95% CI, 0.36 to 0.72) and men (OR, 0.54; 95% CI, 0.42 to 0.70). However, there was insufficient evidence for assessing outcomes at 1 year. • Modifiers of effectiveness: 2 studies (1 good quality, 1 fair) reported subgroup analyses of demographic or clinical factors in women and included a total of 395 patients, of which 167 (32%) were women. 1 good-quality study evaluated the comparative effectiveness of PCI vs. fibrinolysis in patients <65 years of age and ≥65 and found no differences in in-hospital mortality among the treatment groups. 1 fair-quality study evaluated patients ≥80 years of age with STEMI. The study was limited by a small overall size, and it did not find significant differences in outcomes in patients ≥80 years with STEMI undergoing PCI compared with usual (supportive) medical care. • Safety concerns: 2 good-quality studies reported safety concerns in women with STEMI and included a total of 1532 patients, of which 367 (24%) were women. 1 study reported a lower nadir hematocrit in women receiving PCI vs. fibrinolysis but no statistically significant differences in the requirement for blood transfusion. Another study reported the proportion of women with intracranial hemorrhage in women who received PCI vs. accelerated t-PA (0% vs. 4.1%). No studies systematically reported radiation exposure, contrast reactions, access site complications, or stent thrombosis in women with STEMI undergoing PCI.

Table 1. Summary of key findings (continued)

Key Question	Strength of Evidence	Conclusions
KQ 2: Women with UA/NSTEMI (early invasive vs. initial conservative)	Effectiveness of interventions 1. Low (women) and high (men) for short-term (6-month) composite outcomes 2. Low (women and men) for intermediate-term (1-year) composite outcomes 3. Insufficient (women) and low (men) for long-term (5-year) composite outcomes Modifiers of effectiveness Insufficient Safety concerns Insufficient	7 studies (6 good quality, 1 fair) compared early invasive (revascularization via PCI or CABG) with initial conservative therapy for women with UA/NSTEMI and contributed evidence about the comparative effectiveness, modifiers of effectiveness, or safety for these interventions. These studies included a total of 17,930 patients, of which 6084 (34%) were women. • Effectiveness of interventions: A meta-analysis of 2 good-quality studies reporting 6-month composite outcomes (death/MI) suggested a benefit of early invasive compared with initial conservative therapy in women (OR, 0.77; 95% CI, 0.28 to 2.12) that, however, was not statistically significant; early invasive therapy was superior to initial conservative therapy in men at 6 months (OR, 0.65; 95% CI, 0.52 to 0.82; p=0.0002). At 1 year, a meta-analysis of 5 good-quality studies showed that the composite outcome (primarily death/MI) suggested a similar benefit in women who received early invasive therapy (OR, 0.78; 95% CI, 0.54 to 1.12) as well as in men (OR, 0.88; 95% CI, 0.64 to 1.20); however, this was not statistically significant. A meta-analysis of 2 good-quality studies with 5-year followup between early invasive and initial conservative therapy for the composite outcome of death/MI in both sexes suggested a small benefit of initial conservative therapy in women (1.05; 95% CI, 0.81 to 1.35) while suggesting a benefit of early invasive therapy in men (0.91; 95% CI, 0.53 to 1.56). Given the small suggested benefit at 5 years in women, the wide confidence interval crossing 1, and the trend favoring early invasive therapy suggested at earlier time points and across time points in men — we cannot support firm conclusions • Modifiers of effectiveness: 2 good-quality studies comparing initial conservative medical therapy to early invasive therapy with PCI reported a subgroup analysis by risk stratification and included a total of 4030 patients, of which 1439 (36%) were women. These studies revealed conflicting results—one showed no difference in treatment outcomes in the intermediate- and high-risk groups; the other showed a higher event rate in women in the groups with moderate-to-high risk for thrombolysis in myocardial infarction. • Safety concerns: 1 good-quality study (2,220 total patients, 757 [34%] women) reported the harms associated with treatment of UA/NSTEMI by sex group but not the rates of events by treatment group. Bleeding in women undergoing PTCA was higher compared with men (adjusted OR, 3.6; 95% CI, 1.6 to 8.3). However, bleeding related to CABG was similar in women and men, with rates of 12.6% and 15%, respectively. No studies systematically reported radiation exposure, contrast reactions, access site complications, stent thrombosis, or infection in women with UA/NSTEMI comparing early invasive with initial conservative therapy.

Table 1. Summary of key findings (continued)

Key Question	Strength of Evidence	Conclusions
KQ 3: Strategy 1—women with stable angina (revascularization vs. optimal medical therapy)	Effectiveness of interventions 1. With the PCI strategy: Moderate (women) and low (men) for long-term (4- to 5-year) composite outcomes 2. With the CABG strategy: Low (women and men) for long-term (4- to 5-year) composite outcomes 3. With both types of revascularization: Moderate (women) and low (men) for long-term (4- to 5-year) composite outcomes	5 studies (all good quality) compared revascularization (PCI or CABG) with optimal medical therapy for women with stable angina and contributed evidence about the comparative effectiveness, modifiers of effectiveness, or safety for these interventions. These studies included a total of 6851 patients, of which 1285 (19%) were women. Effectiveness of interventions: A meta-analysis of 3 good-quality studies with long-term followup on the composite outcomes (death/MI/revascularization) comparing PCI or CABG with optimal medical therapy showed that revascularization was significantly better than optimal medical therapy in women with stable angina (OR, 0.64; 95% CI, 0.47 to 0.89; p=0.008 for PCI strategy trials; OR, 0.56; 95% CI, 0.32 to 0.96; p=0.04 for CABG strategy trials; and OR, 0.59; 95% CI, 0.43 to 0.81; p=0.001 for either PCI or CABG). However, for men with stable angina, the analysis suggested a small benefit for optimal medical therapy when compared with PCI (OR, 1.03; 95% CI, 0.79 to 1.33). This suggested small benefit however has a wide confidence interval crossing 1 and is not supported by additional time periods or by the evidence in women. Analyses suggested a benefit of CABG (OR, 0.62; 95% CI, 0.31 to 1.24) or either PCI or CABG (OR, 0.71; 95% CI, 0.49 to 1.02) in men with stable angina. These findings were not statistically significant and had very wide confidence intervals.

Table 1. Summary of key findings (continued)

Key Question	Strength of Evidence	Conclusions
		10 studies (8 good quality, 2 fair) compared PCI with CABG in women with stable/unstable angina and contributed evidence about the comparative effectiveness, modifiers of effectiveness, or safety for these interventions. These studies included a total of 6289 patients, of which 1583 (25%) were women.
	Effectiveness of interventions 1. Low (women and men) for short-term (30-day) composite outcomes 2. Low (women and men) for intermediate-term (1-year) composite outcomes 3. Low (women) and high (men) for long-term (>2-year) composite outcomes	Effectiveness of interventions: A meta-analysis of 2 good-quality studies reporting a 30-day death outcome showed no statistically significant difference between PCI and CABG in either men or women. The summary odds ratio in women was 0.68 (95% CI, 0.24 to 1.93) and in men was 1.36 (95% CI, 0.44 to 4.24). The odds ratios suggest a possible sex effect, with PCI showing more benefit in women and CABG showing more benefit in men, but the confidence intervals are too wide to support firm conclusions. For 1-year composite outcomes (death/MI/stroke), a meta-analysis of 2 good-quality studies showed lower events in the CABG group for both sexes, but this benefit was not statistically significant. The summary odds ratio in women was 1.30 (95% CI, 0.69 to 2.45) and in men was 1.19 (95% CI, 0.84 to 1.70). For long-term (>2 years) composite outcomes (death/MI/stroke), a meta-analysis of 4 good-quality studies suggested lower events in the CABG group in women (OR, 1.17; 95% CI, 0.90 to 1.54) although again this did not reach statistical significance; however in men, CABG was significantly better than PCI in lowering cardiovascular events (OR, 1.63; 95% CI, 1.20 to 2.23; p=0.002).
KQ 3: Strategy 2—women with stable/unstable angina (PCI vs. CABG)	Modifiers of effectiveness Insufficient Safety concerns Insufficient	Modifiers of effectiveness: 1 good-quality study evaluated the comparative effectiveness of PCI vs. CABG in diabetic patients with stable/unstable angina. The survival rate at 7 years was similar in diabetic women from both treatment groups. However in diabetic men, those treated with CABG had higher survival than those treated with PCI. Safety concerns: 1 good-quality study reported harms associated with PCI compared with CABG among women with UA/NSTEMI and found that bleeding associated with PCI was higher in women compared with men (OR, 29.4; 95% CI, 5.3 to 500; p=0.001). No studies systematically reported radiation exposure, contrast reactions, access site complications, stent thrombosis or infection, in women with UA/NSTEMI undergoing PCI or CABG.

Abbreviations: CABG = coronary artery bypass grafting; CI = confidence interval; MI = myocardial infarction; NSTEMI = non-ST elevation myocardial infarction; OR = odds ratio; PCI = percutaneous coronary intervention; SOE = strength of evidence; STEMI = ST elevation myocardial infarction; t-PA = tissue plasminogen activator; UA = unstable angina

7

Methods

Overview

Our approach to identifying evidence gaps, prioritizing future research, and developing recommendations for stakeholders is outlined in the following steps. Further detail is provided below.

1. Develop an analytic framework from the original CER in order to understand the clinical and policy context of the review and its initial list of Future Research Needs.
2. Create an initial list of evidence gaps based on the CER organized according to the population, interventions, comparators, and outcomes (PICO) framework.[11]
3. Form a stakeholder group representing appropriate clinician, policymaker, and patient perspectives.
4. Expand the list of evidence gaps based on stakeholder input.
5. Perform an updated review of published literature since the last CER (search last updated in December 2011) and a horizon scan for recently published and ongoing studies that may address the evidence gaps, but which are not included in the current CER.
6. Solicit stakeholder prioritization of the identified research gaps based on the updated literature review.
7. Determine the most appropriate study designs for the highest priority research areas.[12]

Analytic Framework

Figure 1 depicts the Key Questions within the context of the population, interventions, comparators of interest, outcomes, timing, and settings (PICOTS). In general, the figure shows that KQ 1 focuses on the population of women presenting with ST elevation myocardial infarction. KQ 1a considers the effectiveness of optimal medical therapy (i.e., fibrinolytics) versus percutaneous coronary intervention (PCI) on clinical outcomes (i.e., nonfatal MI, death, stroke, repeat revascularization, unstable angina, heart failure, repeat hospitalization, length of hospital stay, angina relief, quality of life, or cognitive effects). KQ 1b considers the modifiers of effectiveness (i.e., age, race, demographic and socioeconomic risk factors; coronary disease risk factors; angiography-specific factors; and hospital characteristics). KQ 1c considers the safety concerns associated with each treatment strategy (e.g., adverse drug reactions, radiation exposure, access site complications, renal dysfunction, anaphylaxis, arrhythmias, stent thrombosis, bleeding, infections). KQ 2 focuses on the population of women presenting with unstable angina or non-ST elevation myocardial infarction. KQ 2a considers the effectiveness of initial conservative therapy versus early invasive therapy (PCI or CABG) on clinical outcomes. KQ 2b considers the associated modifiers of effectiveness, and KQ 2c considers the associated safety concerns. KQ 3 focuses on the population of women presenting with stable angina or unstable angina. KQ 3a considers the effectiveness of two treatment strategies on clinical outcomes: (1) optimal medical therapy versus mechanical revascularization (PCI or CABG) in women with stable angina and (2) PCI versus CABG in women with stable or unstable angina. KQ 3b considers the associated modifiers of effectiveness, and KQ 3c considers the associated safety concerns. The evidence gaps identified for this report fit into the analytic framework as follows: The first gap (with its four subparts) investigates the effects of modifiers on treatment strategies for these three populations and corresponds to KQs 1b, 2b, and 3b; the second, third, and fourth gaps concern the effects of these treatment strategies on the short- and long-term outcomes in all three populations, which corresponds to KQs 1a, 2a, and 3a; and the fifth gap (with its three subparts) looks at adverse effects that may occur due to these treatments and corresponds to KQs 1c, 2c, and 3c.

Figure 1. Analytic framework

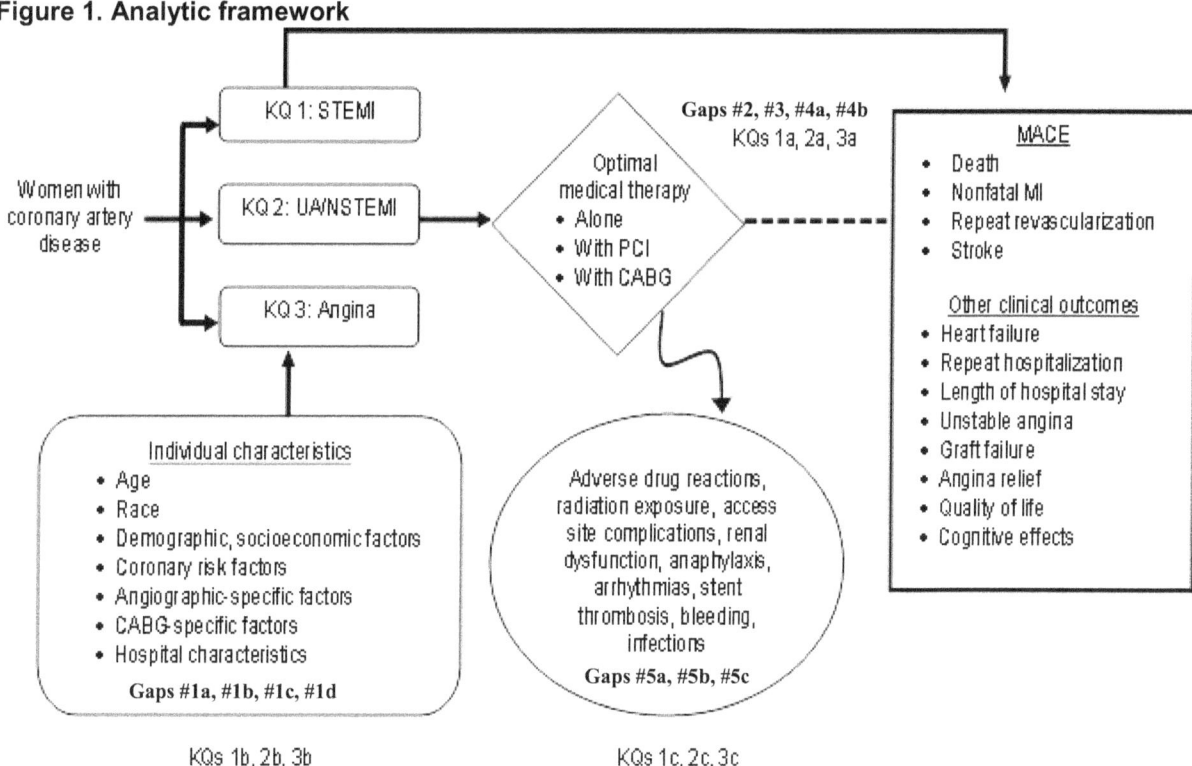

Abbreviations: CABG = coronary artery bypass graft; KQ = Key Question; MACE = major adverse cardiovascular events; MI = myocardial infarction; NSTEMI = non-ST elevation myocardial infarction; PCI = percutaneous coronary intervention; STEMI = ST elevation myocardial infarction; UA/NSTEMI = unstable angina/non-ST elevation myocardial infarction

Initial List of Research Needs

Results from the 2012 report suggest several evidence gaps for future research. These possibilities are neither exhaustive nor prioritized. The initial list generated by the study authors is provided in Table 2, organized according to the PICO format, with the addition of implementation gaps and methods for evidence synthesis.

Table 2. Initial list of evidence gaps

PICO Element	Evidence Gaps
Population	1. Is there evidence that the comparative effectiveness of PCI vs. fibrinolysis/supportive therapy in women with STEMI; early invasive vs. initial conservative therapy in women with UA/NSTEMI; or PCI vs. CABG or revascularization vs. optimal medical therapy in women with stable or unstable angina differs by such characteristics as: a. **Age, race, or other demographic and socioeconomic risk factors?** b. **Coronary disease risk factors** such as diabetes, chronic kidney disease, or other comorbid disease? c. **Angiographic-specific factors** (number of diseased vessels, vessel territory stenoses, left ventricular function, access site, or prior PCI or CABG revascularization procedure)? d. **Hospital characteristics** (hospital volume, setting, guideline-based treatment protocols)?
Intervention and Comparator	2. In women presenting with *STEMI*: What is the effectiveness of PCI vs. fibrinolysis/supportive therapy **on intermediate- or long-term** clinical outcomes (nonfatal MI, death, stroke, repeat revascularization, recurrent unstable angina, heart failure, repeat hospitalization, length of hospital stay, angina relief, quality of life, or cognitive effects)? 3. In women presenting with *UA/NSTEMI*: What is the effectiveness of early invasive (PCI or CABG) vs. initial conservative therapy on **short-, intermediate- or long-term** clinical outcomes (nonfatal MI, death, stroke, repeat revascularization, recurrent unstable angina, heart failure, repeat hospitalization, length of hospital stay, graft failure, angina relief, quality of life, or cognitive effects)? 4. In women presenting with *stable or unstable angina*: What is the effectiveness of the following treatment strategies **on short-, intermediate- or long-term** clinical outcomes (nonfatal MI, death, stroke, repeat revascularization, recurrent unstable angina, heart failure, repeat hospitalization, length of hospital stay, graft failure, angina relief, quality of life, or cognitive effects)? a. Revascularization (PCI or CABG) vs. optimal medical therapy in women with stable angina b. PCI vs. CABG in women with stable or unstable angina
Outcome	5. What are the **potential harms** in women of a. PCI vs. fibrinolysis/supportive therapy with STEMI? b. Early invasive vs. initial conservative therapy with UA/NSTEMI? c. PCI vs. CABG or revascularization vs. optimal medical therapy with stable or unstable angina?

Abbreviations: CABG = coronary artery bypass graft surgery; MI = myocardial infarction; PCI = percutaneous coronary intervention; STEMI = ST elevation myocardial infarction; UA/NSTEMI = unstable angina/non-ST elevation myocardial infarction

Creation of Stakeholder Group

We selected stakeholders to include researchers involved in some of the primary randomized controlled trials (RCTs) included in the CER, other clinical experts and researchers in the content area, representatives from Federal and nongovernmental funding agencies, representatives from relevant professional societies, health care decisionmakers and policymakers, and representatives from related consumer and patient advocacy groups (Table 3). Within each group, we sought to identify an individual who was either familiar with the clinical area and its current uncertainties, or who brought a specific methodological area of expertise to the workgroup.

Table 3. Stakeholder organizations and roles

Organization	Purpose/Role
National Heart, Lung, and Blood Institute	The National Heart, Lung, and Blood Institute is one of the main funders of potential future studies of the comparative safety and effectiveness of treatment strategies for CAD. It will therefore be important to include their perspective in the prioritization of evidence gaps.
American College of Physicians	The American College of Physicians is the largest group representing internal medicine and its subspecialties. A large portion of the care of patients with CAD is managed by generalists or medicine subspecialists in the office setting and the American College of Physicians will represent this broad group of stakeholders.
American College of Cardiology	The American College of Cardiology is comprised of 39,000 cardiovascular specialists, and is a leader in the formulation of health policy, standards, and guidelines for cardiovascular research.
American Heart Association	The American Heart Association funds clinical, outcomes, and health services research in cardiovascular disease and stroke. They are also a leading advocacy group for advancing science and improving the quality of cardiovascular care.
Office of Research on Women's Health	The Office of Research on Women's Health establishes the NIH research agenda for women's health, co-funds research projects in partnership with NIH Institutes and Centers, and ensures that the NIH policy to include women and minorities in clinical research is followed. It will, therefore, be important to include their perspective in the prioritization of evidence gaps.
Payor	We will be seeking a representative from a private payor in the health insurance industry. Although these payors are not likely not be funders of the future research projects, they would be eventual payors of the treatments recommended by the future research studies; and, therefore, their perspective on the types of studies which would be needed to change their coverage decisions would be helpful.
Patient Advocate	We will identify a patient advocate to represent the research priorities and issues from the patient's perspective. This person will be oriented to the topic and relevant issues in advance of the discussion so he/she may be an active participant.
Centers for Medicare and Medicaid Services	We will be seeking a representative from the Centers for Medicare and Medicaid Services. Although the Centers for Medicare and Medicaid Services would not be a funder of the future research projects, they would be eventual payors of the treatments recommended by the future research studies; and, therefore, their perspective on the types of studies which would be needed to change their coverage decisions would be helpful.
Society of Thoracic Surgeons	The Society of Thoracic Surgeons comprises over 6,400 surgeons, researchers, and allied health care professionals dedicated to providing the highest quality of care for patients undergoing cardiothoracic surgery and improving surgical outcomes.

Abbreviations: CAD = coronary artery disease; NIH = National Institutes of Health

We were able to recruit representatives from each of these nine groups. A total of 10 (many representing several of the above perspectives) stakeholders were included in our final panel.

Stakeholder input was solicited and received through web-based survey techniques, email, and group discussions via teleconference. Group discussions were moderated by the Evidence-based Practice Center (EPC) investigators to avoid domination of the discussion by any particular group and to ensure that all participants had an equal opportunity to ask questions and express their views. The AHRQ Task Order Officer was a participant in all group teleconferences and was included on all electronic communication with the stakeholder group.

Each potential stakeholder completed a statement of disclosure, was screened for apparent conflicts of interest, and approved by AHRQ prior to the first stakeholder call. Efforts were made to assemble a balanced group of individuals representing a wide range of perspectives.

Expansion of Research Gaps

We started with the research priorities identified in the CER and input from the stakeholder workgroup during the first call to expand the list of research priorities to include 15 potential evidence gaps (Table 4).

While many of these research areas were within the scope of the initial review, a few raised by the stakeholder group were outside the scope of this review. These areas may represent important gaps in the knowledge base; however, we are less confident about the current state of the evidence since they were not included in the original report. These "out-of-scope" topics were included in our list, but were specifically noted so that the stakeholders were aware that these areas had not undergone the same level of systematic review and we, therefore, could not provide the same level of detail on the state of current evidence.

We have organized these gaps according to the PICO format and listed them Table 4. The areas determined to be out of scope from the original review are italicized in Table 4.

Table 4. Potential Future Research Needs based on the Comparative Effectiveness Review and stakeholder input

PICO Element	Potential Future Research Need
Population	1. Is there evidence that the comparative effectiveness of PCI vs. fibrinolysis/supportive therapy in women with STEMI; early invasive vs. initial conservative therapy in women with UA/NSTEMI; or PCI vs. CABG or revascularization vs. optimal medical therapy in women with stable or unstable angina differs by such characteristics as: **Age, race, or other demographic and socioeconomic risk factors?**
	2. Is there evidence that the comparative effectiveness of PCI vs. fibrinolysis/supportive therapy in women with STEMI; early invasive vs. initial conservative therapy in women with UA/NSTEMI; or PCI vs. CABG or revascularization vs. optimal medical therapy in women with stable or unstable angina differs by such characteristics as: **Coronary disease risk factors such as diabetes, chronic kidney disease, or other comorbid disease?**
	3. Is there evidence that the comparative effectiveness of PCI vs. fibrinolysis/supportive therapy in women with STEMI; early invasive vs. initial conservative therapy in women with UA/NSTEMI; or PCI vs. CABG or revascularization vs. optimal medical therapy in women with stable or unstable angina differs by such characteristics as: **Angiographic-specific factors (number of diseased vessels, vessel territory stenoses, left ventricular function, access site, or prior PCI or CABG revascularization procedure)?**
	4. Is there evidence that the comparative effectiveness of PCI vs. fibrinolysis/supportive therapy in women with STEMI; early invasive vs. initial conservative therapy in women with UA/NSTEMI; or PCI vs. CABG or revascularization vs. optimal medical therapy in women with stable or unstable angina differs by such characteristics as: **Hospital characteristics (hospital volume, setting, guideline-based treatment protocols)?**

Table 4. Potential Future Research Needs based on the Comparative Effectiveness Review and stakeholder input (continued)

PICO Element	Potential Future Research Need
Intervention and comparator	5. In women presenting with **STEMI:** What is the effectiveness of PCI vs. fibrinolysis/supportive therapy on **intermediate- or long-term** clinical outcomes (nonfatal MI, death, stroke, repeat revascularization, recurrent unstable angina, heart failure, repeat hospitalization, length of hospital stay, angina relief, quality of life, or cognitive effects)?
	6. In women presenting with **UA/NSTEMI:** What is the effectiveness of early invasive (PCI or CABG) vs. initial conservative therapy on **short-, intermediate- or long-term** clinical outcomes (nonfatal MI, death, stroke, repeat revascularization, recurrent unstable angina, heart failure, repeat hospitalization, length of hospital stay, graft failure, angina relief, quality of life, or cognitive effects)?
	7. What is the effectiveness of the following treatment strategies on short-, intermediate- or long-term clinical outcomes (nonfatal MI, death, stroke, repeat revascularization, recurrent unstable angina, heart failure, repeat hospitalization, length of hospital stay, graft failure, angina relief, quality of life, or cognitive effects)? **Revascularization (PCI or CABG) vs. optimal medical therapy in women with stable angina**
	8. What is the effectiveness of the following treatment strategies on short-, intermediate- or long-term clinical outcomes (nonfatal MI, death, stroke, repeat revascularization, recurrent unstable angina, heart failure, repeat hospitalization, length of hospital stay, graft failure, angina relief, quality of life, or cognitive effects)? **PCI vs. CABG in women with stable or unstable angina**
	9. Are there gender differences in the instruments used to measure functional status, risk factors, comorbidities, etc. associated with CAD?
Outcome	10. What are the potential harms in women of PCI vs. fibrinolysis/supportive therapy with STEMI?
	11. What are the potential harms in women of early invasive vs. initial conservative therapy with UA/NSTEMI?
	12. What are the potential harms in women of PCI vs. CABG or revascularization vs. optimal medical therapy with stable or unstable angina?
	13. *What are the risks, benefits, and costs of different treatments for CAD, stratified by gender?**
Implementation gaps	14. *Does patient preference or clinician specialty (primary care, cardiology, cardiothoracic surgery) affect the choice of treatment strategy (medical therapy or type of revascularization)?**
	15. *Are the patient outcomes from real-world settings or observational registries similar to the findings from randomized clinical trials?**

Abbreviations: CABG = coronary artery bypass graft surgery; CAD = coronary artery disease; MI = myocardial infarction; PCI = percutaneous coronary intervention; STEMI = ST elevation myocardial infarction; UA/NSTEMI = unstable angina/non-ST elevation myocardial infarction
*Out-of-scope research topics are in italics.

Review of the Current Literature

We performed three database searches to identify ongoing and recently published studies relevant to the identified evidence gaps. These searches included:

1. An update of the PubMed®, Embase, Cochrane Central Registry of Controlled Trials and Cochrane Database of Systematic Reviews searches used in the original CER to identify relevant literature published since the last search date (12/12/2011).

2. A search of PubMed for relevant systematic reviews and meta-analyses included in our original search and in the update which might address the out of scope evidence gaps.

The exact search strategies used are provided in Appendix A.

Search results were reviewed for applicability to the identified research gaps listed in Table 4. We included articles from each search if they met the following criteria: (1) presents original data or secondary analysis of data from an RCT; (2) includes data for between-category comparisons or treatments of interest (optimal medical therapy alone, PCI plus optimal medical therapy, CABG plus optimal medical therapy); (3) Population includes adult women (≥18 years of age) with CAD and angiographically-proven single- or multiple-vessel disease including STEMI, NSTEMI, and stable angina (4) Data for women are reported as a subgroup; and (5) included outcomes that could be categorized according to our identified list of research priorities. The goal for this literature search was to provide the stakeholders with an idea of which research areas had recent or ongoing literature to address these gaps. Since we did not intend to synthesize this data with the existing report, these articles did not undergo full article abstraction or reconciliation of differences between article reviewers. We did, however, review the full-text of the relevant articles as the reporting of gender-specific outcomes was often not clear at the abstract level.

The search of each database yielded the following list of articles:

Updated PubMed®, Embase, Cochrane Central Registry of Controlled Trials and Cochrane Database of Systematic Reviews searches and search of systematic reviews on out of scope topics:

- 613 articles found in updated search
- 46 included as potentially relevant based on abstract screening
- 7 included as relevant based on full text screening

Based on these searches, we created a list of articles and systematic reviews pertaining to the initial list of 15 identified evidence gaps. Relevant literature was identified for four of the 15 initial evidence gaps; that number decreased to three of 14 after the removal of the overarching evidence gap. Of note, the search was unable to identify any articles relevant to the out-of-scope evidence gaps. This document was provided to the stakeholders prior to their final prioritization and is reproduced in Appendix B.

Research Prioritization

Process Used

The stakeholders were provided the AHRQ Effective Health Care Program prioritization criteria for Future Research Needs and instructed to use these criteria (potential value criteria [for significant health impact] for addressing the evidence gaps of knowledge, translation, and implementation) as the basis for their decisions regarding research prioritization.

Potential Value Criteria

- Potential for new knowledge (research would not be redundant; Question not sufficiently researched, including completed and in-process research; Utility of available evidence limited by changes in practice, e.g., disease detection or evolution in technology)

- Potential for significant health impact on the current and future health status of people with respect to burden of the disease and health outcomes: mortality, morbidity, and quality of life.
- Potential to reduce important inappropriate (or unexplained) variation in clinical practices known to relate to quality of care; potential to resolve controversy or dilemmas in what constitutes appropriate health care; potential to improve decisionmaking for patient or provider, by decreasing uncertainty
- Potential for significant (nontrivial) economic impact related to the costs of health service: to reduce unnecessary or excessive costs; to reduce high costs due to high volume use; to reduce high costs due to high unit cost or aggregate cost. Costs may impact consumers, patients, health care systems, or payers.
- Potential risk from inaction: unintended harms from lack of prioritization of proposed research; opportunity cost of inaction
- Addresses inequities and vulnerable and diverse populations (including issues for patient subgroups); potential to reduce health inequities
- Potential to allow assessment of ethical, legal, social issues pertaining to the condition

Probability of Success Criteria

Feasibility
- Feasibility of proposed study duration
- Feasibility of proposed study costs (are costs of study reasonable given overall resource constraints)

Likelihood
- Likelihood that the study would fill an identified evidence gap
- Likelihood that the study would fill an implementation gap (likely to improve translation of research findings or existing recommendations into clinical practice or identify improved strategies for research translation)
- Likelihood that the study question be answered by a study with low risk of bias?
- Likelihood needed result could be produced in timely manner (efficiency)
- Likelihood that study would provide evidence about both health benefits and potential harms
- Likelihood of change (proposed topic exists within a clinical, consumer, or policymaking context that is likely amenable to evidence-based change)

Capacity
- Sufficient research capability and capacity so that the issue can be addressed with confidence
- Utilizes existing resources or builds desired research capacity or decisional support
- Effectively utilizes existing research and knowledge by considering where there is no other research planned or in progress that will answer the research question (nonduplicative)

Participants in our stakeholder group participated in two conference calls, each of which was followed by an online prioritization exercise. The first call (May 2012) was used to introduce the stakeholder group to the project's objective and to describe the key clinical questions, the original CER report and its findings, and the proposed methods for the prioritization process. During this meeting, the identified research priorities were introduced to the stakeholders, and the group was invited to share feedback regarding additional research priorities. Following this conference call, the stakeholders were invited to perform an initial online ranking of the identified research priorities (including the additional priorities identified by the stakeholder team). This ranking utilized a forced-ranking prioritization method, whereby participants were given 5 votes, which could be allocated to any of the 15 research priorities, with a maximum of 3 votes per item.

Stakeholders then participated in a second conference call (July 2012), during which the Duke EPC team shared the search results for relevant ongoing and recently published studies, as well as the stakeholders' initial ranking of research priorities results. During this conference call, the majority of the time was dedicated to discussing prioritization, and it was decided to drop one of the evidence gaps. The group felt that this gap (#13 in Table 4) encompassed all of the others and was preventing the true ranking of the 14 remaining gaps. Following this second call, a final online ranking exercise was distributed to the stakeholder group. This exercise utilized the same prioritization method as the first ranking exercise, and produced the final ranked list of research priorities. Research needs were ranked into tiers; only those in the top tier moved on to the final stage of study design development.

Research Question Development and Research Design Considerations

For the top tier Future Research Needs, we considered advantages and disadvantages of various potential study designs.[12] We adapted a conceptual framework for recommending study designs based on our prior report "Future Research Needs for Angiotensin Converting Enzyme Inhibitors or Angiotensin II Receptor Blockers Added to Standard Medical Therapy for Treating Stable Ischemic Heart Disease."[13] Our overall approach to recommending study designs for addressing specific evidence gaps was to emphasize the study design with the least risk of bias, but the greatest likelihood of completion. For areas outside of the original CER scope, we suggested specific study designs that may be appropriate, while remaining cognizant that without a comprehensive systematic review, one cannot determine with certainty the degree to which those evidence gaps have already been addressed. A thorough systematic review may be the most appropriate initial step before further original research is undertaken for the priorities out of scope from the CER. The figure depicting this framework and a discussion of different designs is included in Appendix C.

Results

Based on the 2012 CER and our discussion with stakeholders, we identified the 15 potential research areas listed in Table 4. Not all areas were considered within the scope of the 2012 CER; these out-of-scope areas are highlighted in italics. Since these areas were out of scope for the original review, it is unclear whether large evidence gaps exist for these areas; however, they were identified and deemed potentially important by the stakeholder panel. During the second stakeholder call, it was decided to remove the research area listed as number 13 in Table 4 (What are the risks, benefits, and costs of different treatments for CAD, stratified by gender?). Both the stakeholders and the EPC team felt that this research area encompassed all other research areas in the list, and for this reason received a score almost twice as high as the next-highest ranked area. Thus, this research area was skewing the rankings because participants were using most of their ranking points on it and had few left for the remaining research areas. In the final stakeholder ranking, 9 of the 10 stakeholders participated and ranked the 14 final research priorities. The final ranking is listed below in Table 5 and is divided into a top, middle, and lower tier, based on the overall score.

Table 5. Final ranking of Future Research Needs for treatment strategies for women with CAD

Tier	Question	Score
Top Tier	What is the effectiveness of the following treatment strategies on short-, intermediate- or long-term clinical outcomes (nonfatal MI, death, stroke, repeat revascularization, recurrent unstable angina, heart failure, repeat hospitalization, length of hospital stay, graft failure, angina relief, quality of life, or cognitive effects)? **Revascularization (PCI or CABG) vs. optimal medical therapy in women with unstable angina**	13
Middle Tier	Is there evidence that the comparative effectiveness of PCI vs. fibrinolysis/supportive therapy in women with STEMI; early invasive vs. initial conservative therapy in women with UA/NSTEMI; or PCI vs. CABG or revascularization vs. optimal medical therapy in women with stable or unstable angina differs by such characteristics as: **Coronary disease risk factors such as diabetes, chronic kidney disease, or other comorbid disease?**	5
	What is the effectiveness of the following treatment strategies on short-, intermediate- or long-term clinical outcomes (nonfatal MI, death, stroke, repeat revascularization, recurrent unstable angina, heart failure, repeat hospitalization, length of hospital stay, graft failure, angina relief, quality of life, or cognitive effects)? **PCI vs. CABG in women with stable or unstable angina**	4
	What are the **potential harms** in women of PCI vs. CABG or revascularization vs. optimal medical therapy with stable or unstable angina?	4
	*Are the **patient outcomes from real-world settings** or observational registries similar to the findings from randomized clinical trials?**	4
	Is there evidence that the comparative effectiveness of PCI vs. fibrinolysis/supportive therapy in women with STEMI; early invasive vs. initial conservative therapy in women with UA/NSTEMI; or PCI vs. CABG or revascularization vs. optimal medical therapy in women with stable or unstable angina differs by such characteristics as: **Angiographic-specific factors (number of diseased vessels, vessel territory stenoses, left ventricular function, access site, or prior PCI or CABG revascularization procedure)?**	3
	*Does **patient preference or clinical specialty** (primary care, cardiology, cardiothoracic surgery) affect the choice of treatment strategy (medical therapy or type of revascularization)?**	3

Table 5. Final ranking of Future Research Needs for treatment strategies for women with CAD (continued)

Tier	Question	Score
Lower Tier	Is there evidence that the comparative effectiveness of PCI vs. fibrinolysis/supportive therapy in women with STEMI; early invasive vs. initial conservative therapy in women with UA/NSTEMI; or PCI vs. CABG or revascularization vs. optimal medical therapy in women with stable or unstable angina differs by such characteristics as: **Age, race, or other demographic and socioeconomic risk factors?**	2
	In women presenting with STEMI: What is the effectiveness **of PCI vs. fibrinolysis/supportive therapy** on intermediate- or long-term clinical outcomes (nonfatal MI, death, stroke, repeat revascularization, recurrent unstable angina, heart failure, repeat hospitalization, length of hospital stay, angina relief, quality of life, or cognitive effects)?	2
	In women presenting with UA/NSTEMI: What is the effectiveness of **early invasive (PCI or CABG) vs. initial conservative therapy** on short-, intermediate- or long-term clinical outcomes (nonfatal MI, death, stroke, repeat revascularization, recurrent unstable angina, heart failure, repeat hospitalization, length of hospital stay, graft failure, angina relief, quality of life, or cognitive effects)?	2
	*Are there **gender differences** in the instruments used to measure functional status, risk factors, comorbidities, etc. associated with CAD?**	2
	What are the **potential harms** in women of early invasive vs. initial conservative therapy with UA/NSTEMI?	2
	Is there evidence that the comparative effectiveness of PCI vs. fibrinolysis/supportive therapy in women with STEMI; early invasive vs. initial conservative therapy in women with UA/NSTEMI; or PCI vs. CABG or revascularization vs. optimal medical therapy in women with stable or unstable angina differs by such characteristics as: **Hospital characteristics** (hospital volume, setting, guideline-based treatment protocols)?	1
	What are **the potential harms** in women of PCI vs. fibrinolysis/supportive therapy with STEMI?	1

Abbreviations: CABG = coronary artery bypass graft surgery; CAD = coronary artery disease; MI = myocardial infarction; PCI = percutaneous coronary intervention; STEMI = ST elevation myocardial infarction; UA/NSTEMI = unstable angina/non-ST elevation myocardial infarction
*Out-of-scope research topics are highlighted in italics.

These final rankings were somewhat changed from the preliminary rankings provided by the stakeholders prior to the second call, as was expected after the removal of the highest-ranked research are from the preliminary exercise. Of note is that no studies were given a score of zero in the second ranking, while there were three studies with a score of zero in the first ranking, indicating that the removal of the overarching evidence gap allowed for a more complete ranking of these three gaps against each other. The second research area in the top tier, which was originally only separated from the next highest gap by two points, became the far and away highest ranked research gap. The remaining 13 gaps were not greatly separated from each other by score, which is similar to the results from the first ranking exercise. Two evidence gaps from the middle tier fell to the lower tier; these were related to angiographic factors affecting treatment type, and the potential harms in women of different treatments for stable and unstable angina. Only one lower tier evidence gap moved up to the middle tier, and its focus was on gender differences in the instrumentation used for CAD. Based on the stakeholder-identified top tier, the EPC team discussed potential study designs for each research area—these are listed in Table 6. While the proposed methods to address each area are not intended to be restrictive of potential study designs, this section is intended to discuss the benefits or limitations for each study design for answering these questions.

Table 6. High-priority research area and possible study designs

Research Area	RCT?	Meta-Analysis or Individual Patient Data Analysis Across RCTs?	Meta-Analysis of Observational Studies?	New Observational Study?	Analysis of Existing Data?	Model?
What is the effectiveness of the following treatment strategies on short-, intermediate- or long-term clinical outcomes (nonfatal MI, death, stroke, repeat revascularization, recurrent unstable angina, heart failure, repeat hospitalization, length of hospital stay, graft failure, angina relief, quality of life, or cognitive effects)? **Revascularization (PCI or CABG) vs. optimal medical therapy in women with stable angina**	**Yes:** RCT with women only or large enough sample size with stratification of randomization by sex to allow for meaningful sex-based analyses would provide most informative evidence	**Maybe:** Maybe appropriate if sufficient studies, including those studies that did not report sex-stratified outcomes	**Yes:** if the individual patient data is available from the observational studies and the short-, intermediate-, and long-term outcomes are ascertained the same way for the different treatment strategies	**Maybe:** if RCT is not feasible, then an observational study could explore the evidence gap though without the same fidelity	**No:** Unlikely to help as very few comparative studies currently exist with short-, intermediate, or long-term clinical outcomes for women with stable angina	**Maybe:** Potential role for helping determine clinically important differences

Abbreviations: CABG = coronary artery bypass graft surgery; MI = myocardial infarction; PCI = percutaneous coronary intervention; RCT = randomized controlled trial; STEMI = ST elevation myocardial infarction; UA/NSTEMI = unstable angina/non-ST elevation myocardial infarction

19

Discussion

The 2012 CER, "Treatment Strategies for Women With Coronary Artery Disease,"[10] assessed the comparative effectiveness of treatment options for women with CAD. However, there was low or insufficient evidence from comparative studies to clearly describe short, intermediate, or long-term clinical outcomes of different treatment strategies on women presenting with different forms of coronary artery disease due to the small numbers of women recruited for these clinical trials. Also, there was insufficient evidence to describe the clinical outcomes of different treatment strategies for women with different cardiovascular risk factors, such as diabetes, chronic kidney disease, or other comorbid disease. The recommendations for future research on treatment strategies for women with CAD found in this report represent a broad range of stakeholder perspectives including those of general physicians, physician specialists, researchers, policymakers, and patients. The prioritized areas represent two primary foci: (1) clinical decisionmaking (i.e., the effect of treatment decisions on clinical outcomes); and (2) implementation and generalizability (i.e., the effect of risk factors and comorbid disease on treatment outcomes).

Determining the best treatment strategy in women presenting with different forms of coronary artery disease is critically important given that coronary artery disease is the number one cause of death among women. Future clinical trials to determine long-term clinical outcomes for different presentations of CAD and with different treatment strategies should be designed with recruitment of only women or with recruitment of large enough sample sizes with stratification of randomization by sex to allow for meaningful sex-based analyses. While the most preferable data on clinical outcomes by CAD presentation and treatment strategy would come from new clinical trials, meta-analyses of existing data could contribute to our knowledge in this area. Our review excluded trials that looked for a sex effect yet failed to provide results of women and men by treatment arm. Meta-analyses of existing trials, including those that we excluded, could be performed if patient level data were available in order to stratify treatment and outcomes by sex.

Knowing the influence of different clinical factors on cardiovascular outcomes is important for determining the proper treatment strategy and prognosis of women patients who present with various risk factors and comorbidities. Based on the small number of studies that looked at demographic and clinical factors that influence response to treatment strategies in women, there was insufficient evidence that clinicians can use to determine if certain coronary risk factors should be given greater consideration when deciding on a treatment strategy for women with CAD. It would be difficult to design clinical trials to compare the influence of these different clinical factors on response to treatment strategy. Prospective, observational studies, however, could be designed with standardized and clearly defined treatment strategies and clinical outcomes. These databases could then be used to compare outcomes among women with different clinical risk factors.

Given the limited time the stakeholders have to review the existing evidence, it is also possible that their prioritization represents their general research priorities, rather than the state of evidence for this specific topic. The observation that the top-ranked research priorities focus on the general population of women with CAD, while the majority of research priorities in the lower tier focus on specific populations (women with STEMI or UA/NSTEMI), may be a reflection of this. The CER on this topic noted the lack of evidence due to low numbers of enrollment of women presenting with different forms of CAD, yet not all stakeholders are concerned with these subtypes. It is interesting to note as well that the initial and final top-ranked research priorities were scored so much higher than the next-ranked priority, and that the final top-ranked priority more than doubled its score between the first and second ranking exercises. As AHRQ prepares further prioritization reports, it would be interesting to examine recurrent themes that arise in the top tier of research priorities since they are of direct interest to researchers in the field.

The stakeholder group included a few topics that were out-of-scope for the original review. These topics are related to issues occurring in actual practice, such as the effects of real-world settings and clinician specialty on patient outcomes. While the original search strategy may have identified studies addressing these topics, these outcomes were not part of the outcomes of interest in the CER and so there is no available summary of the strength of evidence. The expansion of topics promotes consideration of new areas of research that have not been adequately explored, and this is evidenced by the literature scan in this report, which was unable to identify any articles of relevance to these out-of-scope topics. Nevertheless, the original CER did not comment on the state of current research in these out-of-scope areas, and they should only be promoted with the caveat that existing literature may already adequately address these areas.

Conclusions

A workgroup of 10 stakeholders (9 completing the online rankings) identified the following research area as by far the highest priority for future research for the comparative effectiveness of treatment strategies for women with CAD.

1. What is the effectiveness of the following treatment strategies on short-, intermediate- or long-term clinical outcomes (i.e., nonfatal MI, death, stroke, repeat revascularization, recurrent unstable angina, heart failure, repeat hospitalization, length of hospital stay, graft failure, angina relief, quality of life, or cognitive effects)? **Revascularization (PCI or CABG) versus optimal medical therapy in women with unstable angina**

    a. Recommended study design: (preferable) large long-term clinical trial with women-only enrollment or of large enough sample size with stratification of randomization by sex to allow for meaningful sex-based analyses; also possible would be meta-analyses of all existing clinical trials with patient-level data to more accurately describe sex-stratified outcomes

References

1. Roger VL, Go AS, Lloyd-Jones DM, et al. Heart Disease and Stroke Statistics--2012 Update: A Report From the American Heart Association. Circulation. 2012 Jan 3;125(1):e2-e220. PMID: 22179539.

2. Mosca L, Banka CL, Benjamin EJ, et al. Evidence-based guidelines for cardiovascular disease prevention in women: 2007 update. Circulation. 2007 Mar 20;115(11):1481-501. PMID: 17309915.

3. Shaw LJ, Bugiardini R, Merz CN. Women and ischemic heart disease: evolving knowledge. J Am Coll Cardiol. 2009 Oct 20;54(17):1561-75. PMID: 19833255.

4. Hochman JS, Tamis JE, Thompson TD, et al. Sex, clinical presentation, and outcome in patients with acute coronary syndromes. Global Use of Strategies to Open Occluded Coronary Arteries in Acute Coronary Syndromes IIb Investigators. N Engl J Med. 1999 July 22;341(4):226-32. PMID: 10413734.

5. Berger JS, Elliott L, Gallup D, et al. Sex differences in mortality following acute coronary syndromes. JAMA. 2009 Aug 26;302(8):874-82. PMID: 19706861.

6. Mieres JH, Shaw LJ, Arai A, et al. Role of noninvasive testing in the clinical evaluation of women with suspected coronary artery disease: consensus statement from the Cardiac Imaging Committee, Council on Clinical Cardiology, and the Cardiovascular Imaging and Intervention Committee, Council on Cardiovascular Radiology and Intervention, American Heart Association. Circulation. 2005 Feb 8;111(5):682-96. PMID: 15687114.

7. Alexander KP, Chen AY, Newby LK, et al. Sex differences in major bleeding with glycoprotein IIb/IIIa inhibitors: results from the CRUSADE (Can Rapid risk stratification of Unstable angina patients Suppress ADverse outcomes with Early implementation of the ACC/AHA guidelines) initiative. 2006 Sep 26;114(13):1380-7. PMID: 16982940.

8. Pepine CJ. Ischemic heart disease in women: facts and wishful thinking. 2004 May 19;43(10):1727-30. PMID: 15145090.

9. Vaccarino V, Abramson JL, Veledar E, et al. Sex differences in hospital mortality after coronary artery bypass surgery: evidence for a higher mortality in younger women. Circulation. 2002 Mar 12;105(10):1176-81. PMID: 11889010.

10. Dolor RJ, Melloni C, Chatterjee R, et al. Treatment Strategies for Women With Coronary Artery Disease. Comparative Effectiveness Review No. 66. (Prepared by the Duke Evidence-based Practice Center under Contract No. 290-2007-10066-I.) AHRQ Publication No. 12-EHC070-EF. Rockville, MD: Agency for Healthcare Research and Quality. August 2012. www.effectivehealthcare.ahrq.gov/reports/final.cfm.

11. Robinson KA, Saldanha IJ, McKoy NA. Development of a framework to identify research gaps from systematic reviews. J Clin Epidemiol 2011 Dec;64(12):1325-30. PMID: 21937195.

12. Carey T, Sanders GD, Viswanathan M, et al. Framework for Considering Study Designs for Future Research Needs. Methods Future Research Needs Paper No. 8. (Prepared by the RTI–UNC Evidence-based Practice Center under Contract No. 290-2007-10056-I.) AHRQ Publication No. 12-EHC048-EF. Rockville, MD: Agency for Healthcare Research and Quality. March 2012. www.effectivehealthcare.ahrq.gov/reports/final.cfm.

13. Sanders GD, Powers B, Crowley M, et al. Future Research Needs for Angiotensin Converting Enzyme Inhibitors or Angiotensin II Receptor Blockers Added to Standard Medical Therapy for Treating Stable Ischemic Heart Disease. Future Research Needs Paper No. 8. (Prepared by Duke Evidence-based Practice Center under Contract No. 290-2007-10066-I.) AHRQ Publication No. 11-EHC006-EF. Rockville, MD: Agency for Healthcare Research and Quality. November 2010. www.effectivehealthcare.ahrq.gov/reports/final.cfm.

Abbreviations

AHRQ	Agency for Healthcare Research and Quality
CABG	Coronary artery bypass graft surgery
CAD	Coronary artery disease
CER	Comparative Effectiveness Review
CI	Confidence interval
EPC	Evidence-based Practice Center
KQ	Key Question
MI	Myocardial infarction
NSTEMI	Non-ST elevation myocardial infarction
OR	Odds ratio
PCI	Percutaneous coronary intervention
PICO	Population, interventions, comparators, and outcomes
PICOTS	Population, interventions, comparators, outcomes, timing, and setting
RCT	Randomized controlled trial
SOE	Strength of evidence
STEMI	ST elevation myocardial infarction
UA/NSTEMI	Unstable angina or non-ST elevation myocardial infarction

Appendix A. Exact Search Strings

The exact search strings used for this project are given below.

PubMed® Search Strategy (Update of Search Performed for Original CER)

Search Date: June 4, 2012

Set #	Terms
#1	("cardiovascular diseases"[MeSH Terms] OR ("cardiovascular"[All Fields] AND "diseases"[All Fields]) OR "cardiovascular diseases"[All Fields]) OR ("heart diseases"[MeSH Terms] OR ("heart"[All Fields] AND "diseases"[All Fields]) OR "heart diseases"[All Fields]) OR ("heart"[MeSH Terms] OR "heart"[All Fields] OR "coronary"[All Fields]) OR cardiovas*[All fields] OR cardiac*[All fields] OR ("myocardium"[MeSH Terms] OR "myocardium"[All Fields] OR "myocardial"[All Fields]) OR ("acute coronary syndrome"[MeSH Terms] OR ("acute"[All Fields] AND "coronary"[All Fields] AND "syndrome"[All Fields]) OR "acute coronary syndrome"[All Fields]) OR ("myocardial infarction"[MeSH Terms] OR ("myocardial"[All Fields] AND "infarction"[All Fields]) OR "myocardial infarction"[All Fields]) OR ("angina, unstable"[MeSH Terms] OR ("angina"[All Fields] AND "unstable"[All Fields]) OR "unstable angina"[All Fields] OR ("unstable"[All Fields] AND "angina"[All Fields]))
#2	"angioplasty, balloon, coronary"[MeSH Terms] OR ("angioplasty"[All Fields] AND "balloon"[All Fields] AND "coronary"[All Fields]) OR "coronary balloon angioplasty"[All Fields] OR ("percutaneous"[All Fields] AND "transluminal"[All Fields] AND "coronary"[All Fields] AND "angioplasty"[All Fields]) OR "percutaneous transluminal coronary angioplasty"[All Fields] OR "ptca"[All Fields] OR percutaneous coronary intervention[All Fields] OR percutaneous coronary interventional[All Fields] OR percutaneous coronary interventions[All Fields] OR PCI[All Fields] OR stent[All Fields] OR stents[All Fields] OR stent*[All Fields] OR "stents"[MeSH Terms] OR ("balloon"[All Fields] AND "angioplasty"[All Fields]) OR "balloon angioplasty"[All Fields] OR "angioplasty, balloon"[MeSH Terms] OR "balloon dilation"[MeSH Terms] OR ("balloon"[All Fields] AND "dilation"[All Fields]) OR "balloon dilation"[All Fields] OR ("balloon"[All Fields] AND "dilatation"[All Fields]) OR "balloon dilatation"[All Fields] OR ("transluminal"[All Fields] AND "angioplasty"[All Fields]) OR "transluminal angioplasty"[All Fields] OR "angioplasty"[MeSH Terms] OR "angioplasty"[All Fields] OR "atherectomy, coronary"[MeSH Terms] OR ("atherectomy"[All Fields] AND "coronary"[All Fields]) OR "coronary atherectomy"[All Fields] OR ("coronary"[All Fields] AND "atherectomy"[All Fields]) OR ("coronary artery bypass"[MeSH Terms] OR ("coronary"[All Fields] AND "artery"[All Fields] AND "bypass"[All Fields]) OR "coronary artery bypass"[All Fields]) OR CABG[All Fields] OR ("coronary artery bypass"[MeSH Terms] OR ("aortocoronary"[All Fields] AND "bypass"[All Fields]) OR "aortocoronary bypass"[All Fields]) OR "coronary revascularization"[All Fields] OR "myocardial revascularization"[All Fields]
#3	"women"[MeSH Terms] OR "women"[All Fields] OR "woman"[All Fields] OR "female"[MeSH Terms] OR "female"[All Fields] OR "females"[All Fields] OR "sex factors"[MeSH Terms] OR ("sex"[All Fields] AND "factors"[All Fields]) OR "sex factors"[All Fields]
#4	randomized controlled trial[pt] OR controlled clinical trial[pt] OR randomized[tiab] OR placebo[tiab] OR "clinical trials as topic"[MeSH Terms:noexp] OR randomly[tiab] OR trial[ti]
#5	#1 AND #2 AND #3 AND #4
#6	#5 NOT (Editorial[ptyp] OR Letter[ptyp] OR Case Reports[ptyp]) NOT Animals[Mesh:noexp]
	Limits: Human, English, Publication Date: 2001- Present

Embase® Search Strategy (Update of Search Performed for Original CER)

Platform: Embase.com

Search Date: June 4, 2012

Set #	Terms
#1	'cardiovascular disease'/exp OR 'heart disease'/exp OR 'heart'/exp OR 'acute coronary syndrome'/exp OR 'heart infarction'/exp OR 'unstable angina pectoris'/exp OR 'cardiovascular diseases':ab OR 'heart diseases':ab OR heart:ab OR cardiovasc*:ab OR cardiac*:ab OR coronary:ab OR myocardial:ab OR 'acute coronary syndrome':ab OR 'myocardial infarction':ab OR 'unstable angina':ab OR 'cardiovascular diseases':ti OR 'heart diseases':ti OR heart:ti OR cardiovasc*:ti OR cardiac*:ti OR coronary:ti OR myocardial:ti OR 'acute coronary syndrome':ti OR 'myocardial infarction':ti OR 'unstable angina':ti
#2	'transluminal coronary angioplasty'/exp OR 'percutaneous coronary intervention'/exp OR 'stent'/exp OR 'balloon dilatation'/exp OR 'percutaneous transluminal angioplasty'/exp OR 'atherectomy'/exp OR 'percutaneous transluminal angioplasty':ti OR ptca:ti OR ('percutaneous coronary' NEXT/1 intervention*):ti OR pci:ti OR stent*:ti OR 'balloon angioplasty':ti OR 'balloon dilation':ti OR 'balloon dilatation':ti OR 'transluminal angioplasty':ti OR 'coronary atherectomy':ti OR 'percutaneous transluminal angioplasty':ab OR ptca:ab OR ('percutaneous coronary' NEXT/1 intervention*):ab OR pci:ab OR stent*:ab OR 'balloon angioplasty':ab OR 'balloon dilation':ab OR 'balloon dilatation':ab OR 'transluminal angioplasty':ab OR 'coronary atherectomy':ab OR 'coronary artery bypass graft'/exp OR 'heart muscle revascularization'/exp OR 'coronary artery bypass':ti OR cabg:ti OR 'aortocoronary bypass':ti OR 'coronary revascularization':ti OR 'myocardial revascularization':ti OR 'coronary artery bypass':ab OR cabg:ab OR 'aortocoronary bypass':ab OR 'coronary revascularization':ab OR 'myocardial revascularization':ab OR 'coronary artery recanalization'/exp
#3	'female'/exp OR female OR women OR woman OR females OR 'sex difference'/exp
#4	'randomized controlled trial'/exp OR 'crossover procedure'/exp OR 'double blind procedure'/exp OR 'single blind procedure'/exp OR random* OR factorial* OR crossover* OR cross NEAR/1 over* OR placebo* OR doubl* NEAR/1 blind* OR singl* NEAR/1 blind* OR assign* OR allocat* OR volunteer*
#5	#1 AND #2 AND #3 AND #4
#6	#5 (AND [embase]/lim NOT [medline]/lim)
	Limits: Human, English, Publication Date: 2001- Present

Cochrane Search Strategy (Update of Search Performed for Original CER)

Platform: Wiley
Databases searched: Cochrane Central Registry of Controlled Trials and Cochrane Database of Systematic Reviews

----

Search Date: June 5, 2012

Set #	Terms
#1	cardiovascular diseases OR heart diseases OR heart OR cardiovas* OR cardiac* OR coronary OR myocardial OR acute coronary syndrome OR myocardial infarction OR unstable angina [in title-abstract-keywords]
#2	percutaneous transluminal coronary angioplasty OR PTCA OR "percutaneous coronary intervention" OR "percutaneous coronary interventions" OR "percutaneous coronary interventional" OR PCI OR Stent* OR stents OR Balloon angioplasty OR Balloon dilatation OR Balloon dilation OR Transluminal angioplasty OR coronary atherectomy OR Coronary Artery Bypass OR CABG OR aortocoronary bypass OR coronary revascularization OR myocardial revascularization [in title-abstract-keywords]
#3	women OR woman OR female OR females OR sex factors [in title-abstract-keywords]
#4	#1 AND #2 AND #3
	Limits: 2001- Present

PubMed® Search Strategy (Search for Systematic Reviews)

Search Date: June 5, 2012

Set #	Terms
#1	("cardiovascular diseases"[MeSH Terms] OR ("cardiovascular"[All Fields] AND "diseases"[All Fields]) OR "cardiovascular diseases"[All Fields]) OR ("heart diseases"[MeSH Terms] OR ("heart"[All Fields] AND "diseases"[All Fields]) OR "heart diseases"[All Fields]) OR ("heart"[MeSH Terms] OR "heart"[All Fields] OR "coronary"[All Fields]) OR cardiovas*[All fields] OR cardiac*[All fields] OR ("myocardium"[MeSH Terms] OR "myocardium"[All Fields] OR "myocardial"[All Fields]) OR ("acute coronary syndrome"[MeSH Terms] OR ("acute"[All Fields] AND "coronary"[All Fields] AND "syndrome"[All Fields]) OR "acute coronary syndrome"[All Fields]) OR ("myocardial infarction"[MeSH Terms] OR ("myocardial"[All Fields] AND "infarction"[All Fields]) OR "myocardial infarction"[All Fields]) OR ("angina, unstable"[MeSH Terms] OR ("angina"[All Fields] AND "unstable"[All Fields]) OR "unstable angina"[All Fields] OR ("unstable"[All Fields] AND "angina"[All Fields]))
#2	"angioplasty, balloon, coronary"[MeSH Terms] OR ("angioplasty"[All Fields] AND "balloon"[All Fields] AND "coronary"[All Fields]) OR "coronary balloon angioplasty"[All Fields] OR ("percutaneous"[All Fields] AND "transluminal"[All Fields] AND "coronary"[All Fields] AND "angioplasty"[All Fields]) OR "percutaneous transluminal coronary angioplasty"[All Fields] OR "ptca"[All Fields] OR percutaneous coronary intervention[All Fields] OR percutaneous coronary interventional[All Fields] OR percutaneous coronary interventions[All Fields] OR PCI[All Fields] OR stent[All Fields] OR stents[All Fields] OR stent*[All Fields] OR "stents"[MeSH Terms] OR ("balloon"[All Fields] AND "angioplasty"[All Fields]) OR "balloon angioplasty"[All Fields] OR "angioplasty, balloon"[MeSH Terms] OR "balloon dilation"[MeSH Terms] OR ("balloon"[All Fields] AND "dilation"[All Fields]) OR "balloon dilation"[All Fields] OR ("balloon"[All Fields] AND "dilatation"[All Fields]) OR "balloon dilatation"[All Fields] OR ("transluminal"[All Fields] AND "angioplasty"[All Fields]) OR "transluminal angioplasty"[All Fields] OR "angioplasty"[MeSH Terms] OR "angioplasty"[All Fields] OR "atherectomy, coronary"[MeSH Terms] OR ("atherectomy"[All Fields] AND "coronary"[All Fields]) OR "coronary atherectomy"[All Fields] OR ("coronary"[All Fields] AND "atherectomy"[All Fields]) OR ("coronary artery bypass"[MeSH Terms] OR ("coronary"[All Fields] AND "artery"[All Fields] AND "bypass"[All Fields]) OR "coronary artery bypass"[All Fields]) OR CABG[All Fields] OR ("coronary artery bypass"[MeSH Terms] OR ("aortocoronary"[All Fields] AND "bypass"[All Fields]) OR "aortocoronary bypass"[All Fields]) OR "coronary revascularization"[All Fields] OR "myocardial revascularization"[All Fields]
#3	"women"[MeSH Terms] OR "women"[All Fields] OR "woman"[All Fields] OR "female"[MeSH Terms] OR "female"[All Fields] OR "females"[All Fields] OR "sex factors"[MeSH Terms] OR ("sex"[All Fields] AND "factors"[All Fields]) OR "sex factors"[All Fields] OR gender[tiab]
#4	"Patient Preference"[Mesh] OR prefer[tiab] OR preferred[tiab] OR preference[tiab] OR "Cardiology"[Mesh] OR cardiology[tiab] OR cardiologist[tiab] OR specialist[tiab] OR specialty[tiab] OR "Primary Health Care"[Mesh] OR "Physicians, Primary Care"[Mesh] OR "primary care"[tiab] cardiothoracic[tiab] OR "Decision Making"[Mesh] OR decision[tiab] OR decide[tiab] OR decided[tiab] OR choice[tiab] OR "Economics"[Mesh] OR "economics" [Subheading] OR cost[tiab] OR costs[tiab]
#5	#1 AND #2 AND #3 AND #4
#6	#5 AND systematic[subset] OR "meta-analysis"[Publication Type] OR "meta-analysis as topic"[MeSH Terms] OR "meta-analysis"[tw] OR "meta-analyses"[tw]) NOT (Editorial[ptyp] OR Letter[ptyp] OR Case Reports[ptyp] OR Comment[ptyp]) NOT (animals[mh] NOT humans[mh])
	Limits: English, Publication Date: 2005-

Appendix B. Table of Research Priorities Linked to Recent Publications and Ongoing Studies

Priority	Details
1	What is the effectiveness of the following treatment strategies on short-, intermediate- or long-term clinical outcomes (nonfatal MI, death, stroke, repeat revascularization, recurrent unstable angina, heart failure, repeat hospitalization, length of hospital stay, graft failure, angina relief, quality of life, or cognitive effects)? <u>Revascularization (PCI or CABG) versus optimal medical therapy in women with stable angina</u> MEDLINE/Embase/Cochrane: **No relevant citations found**
2	Is there evidence that the comparative effectiveness of PCI versus fibrinolysis/supportive therapy in women with STEMI; early invasive versus initial conservative therapy in women with UA/NSTEMI; or PCI versus CABG or revascularization versus optimal medical therapy in women with stable or unstable angina differs by such characteristics as: <u>Coronary disease risk factors such as diabetes, chronic kidney disease, or other comorbid disease?</u> MEDLINE/Embase/Cochrane: No relevant citations found
3	What is the effectiveness of the following treatment strategies on short-, intermediate- or long-term clinical outcomes (nonfatal MI, death, stroke, repeat revascularization, recurrent unstable angina, heart failure, repeat hospitalization, length of hospital stay, graft failure, angina relief, quality of life, or cognitive effects)? <u>PCI versus CABG in women with stable or unstable angina</u> **MEDLINE/Embase/Cochrane:** Manfrini O, Eskola M, Karhunen P, et al. Coronary revascularization in patients that become stable. J Am Coll Cardiol. 2012;59(13):E363. Hlatky MA, Boothroyd DB, Bravata DM, et al. Coronary artery bypass surgery compared with percutaneous coronary interventions for multivessel disease: a collaborative analysis of individual patient data from ten randomised trials. Lancet. 2009;373(9670):1190-7.
4	What are the potential harms in women of PCI versus CABG or revascularization versus optimal medical therapy with stable or unstable angina? MEDLINE/Embase/Cochrane: No relevant citations found
5	Are the patient outcomes from real-world settings or observational registries similar to the findings from randomized clinical trials? MEDLINE/Embase/Cochrane: No relevant citations found
6	Is there evidence that the comparative effectiveness of PCI versus fibrinolysis/supportive therapy in women with STEMI; early invasive versus initial conservative therapy in women with UA/NSTEMI; or PCI versus CABG or revascularization versus optimal medical therapy in women with stable or unstable angina differs by such characteristics as: <u>Angiographic-specific factors (number of diseased vessels, vessel territory stenoses, left ventricular function, access site, or prior PCI or CABG revascularization procedure)?</u> MEDLINE/Embase/Cochrane: No relevant citations found
7	Does patient preference or clinician specialty (primary care, cardiology, cardiothoracic surgery) affect the choice of treatment strategy (medical therapy or type of revascularization)? MEDLINE/Embase/Cochrane: No relevant citations found
8	Is there evidence that the comparative effectiveness of PCI versus fibrinolysis/supportive therapy in women with STEMI; early invasive versus initial conservative therapy in women with UA/NSTEMI; or PCI versus CABG or revascularization versus optimal medical therapy in women with stable or unstable angina differs by such characteristics as: <u>Age, race, or other demographic and socioeconomic risk factors?</u> MEDLINE/Embase/Cochrane: No relevant citations found

Priority	Details
9	**In women presenting with ST elevation myocardial infarction (STEMI): What is the effectiveness of percutaneous coronary intervention (PCI) versus fibrinolysis/supportive therapy on intermediate- or long-term clinical outcomes (nonfatal MI, death, stroke, repeat revascularization, recurrent unstable angina, heart failure, repeat hospitalization, length of hospital stay, angina relief, quality of life, or cognitive effects)?** **MEDLINE/Embase/Cochrane:** Reynolds HR, Forman SA, Tamis-Holland JE, et al. Relationship of female sex to outcomes after myocardial infarction with persistent total occlusion of the infarct artery: analysis of the Occluded Artery Trial (OAT). Am Heart J. 2012;163(3):462-9. Yan AT, Yan RT, Mehta SR, et al. Efficacy of early invasive management postfibrinolysis in men versus women with ST-elevation myocardial infarction: A subgroup analysis from transfer-AMI. Canadian Journal of Cardiology. 2011;27(5):S152-S153.
10	**In women presenting with unstable angina or non-ST elevation myocardial infarction (UA/NSTEMI): What is the effectiveness of early invasive (PCI or CABG) versus initial conservative therapy on short-, intermediate- or long-term clinical outcomes (nonfatal MI, death, stroke, repeat revascularization, recurrent unstable angina, heart failure, repeat hospitalization, length of hospital stay, graft failure, angina relief, quality of life, or cognitive effects)?** **MEDLINE/Embase/Cochrane:** Reynolds HR, Forman SA, Tamis-Holland JE, et al. Relationship of female sex to outcomes after myocardial infarction with persistent total occlusion of the infarct artery: analysis of the Occluded Artery Trial (OAT). Am Heart J. 2012;163(3):462-9. Swahn E, Alfredsson J, Afzal R, et al. Early invasive compared with a selective invasive strategy in women with non-ST-elevation acute coronary syndromes: a substudy of the OASIS 5 trial and a meta-analysis of previous randomized trials. Eur Heart J. 2012;33(1):51-60. Kleopatra K, Muth K, Zahn R, et al. Effect of an invasive strategy on in-hospital outcome and one-year mortality in women with non-ST-elevation myocardial infarction. International Journal of Cardiology. 2011;153(3):291-295.
11	**Are there gender differences in the instruments used to measure functional status, risk factors, comorbidities, etc. associated with CAD?** **MEDLINE/Embase/Cochrane:** No relevant citations found
12	**What are the potential harms in women of early invasive versus initial conservative therapy with UA/NSTEMI?** **MEDLINE/Embase/Cochrane:** No relevant citations found
13	**Is there evidence that the comparative effectiveness of PCI versus fibrinolysis/supportive therapy in women with STEMI; early invasive versus initial conservative therapy in women with UA/NSTEMI; or PCI versus CABG or revascularization versus optimal medical therapy in women with stable or unstable angina differs by such characteristics as: Hospital characteristics (hospital volume, setting, guideline-based treatment protocols)?** **MEDLINE/Embase/Cochrane:** No relevant citations found
14	**What are the potential harms in women of PCI vs. fibrinolysis/supportive therapy with STEMI?** **MEDLINE/Embase/Cochrane:** No relevant citations found
Removed prior to 2nd survey	
N/A	**What are the risks, benefits, and costs of different treatments for CAD, stratified by gender?** **MEDLINE/Embase/Cochrane:** Cohen DJ, Lavelle TA, Van Hout B, et al. Economic outcomes of percutaneous coronary intervention with drug-eluting stents versus bypass surgery for patients with left main or three-vessel coronary artery disease: One-year results from the SYNTAX trial. Catheterization and Cardiovascular Interventions. 2012;79(2):198-209.

Appendix C. Criteria for Research Prioritization

Appendix C Figure. Framework for suggesting study designs for Future Research Needs

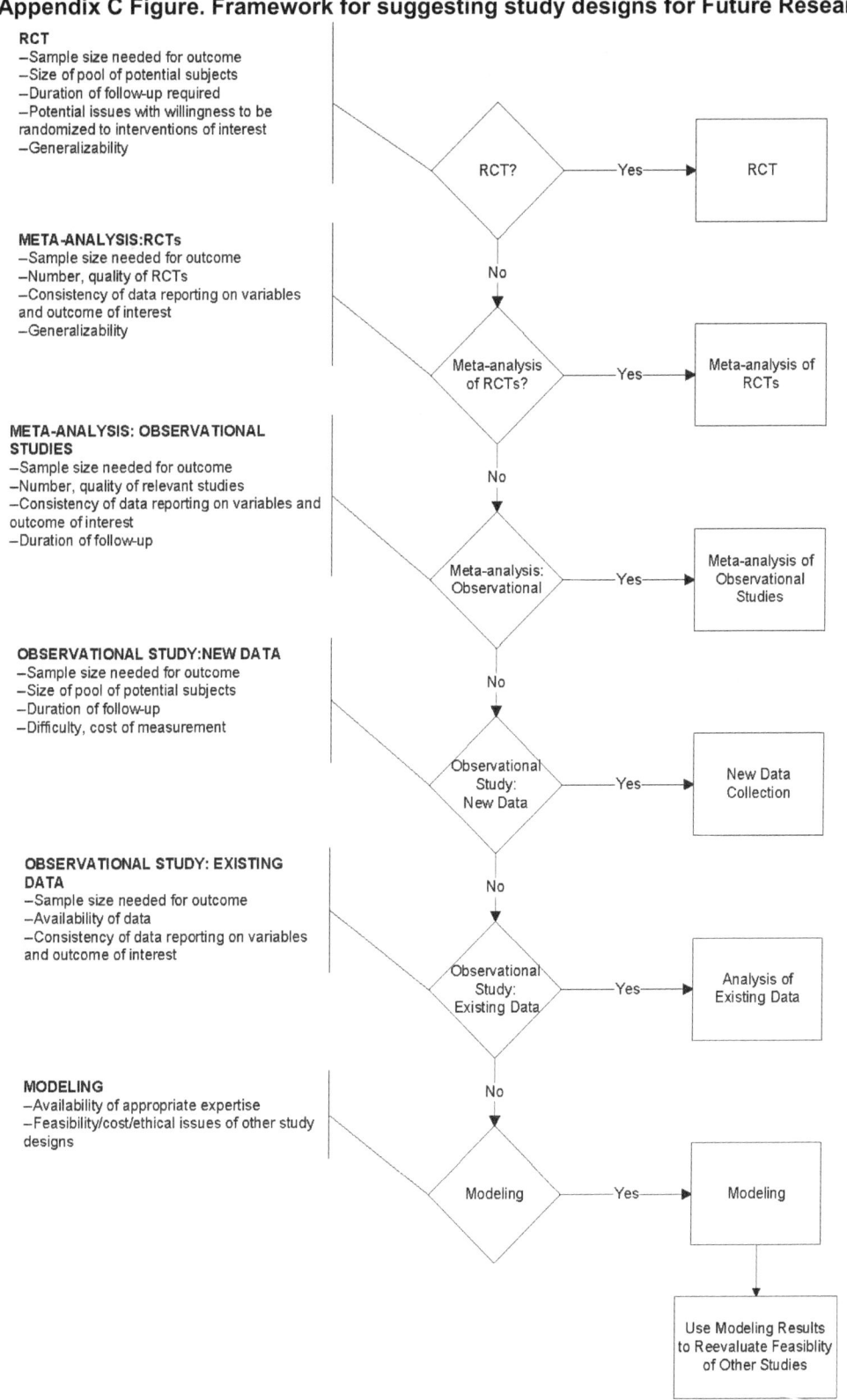

RCT
−Sample size needed for outcome
−Size of pool of potential subjects
−Duration of follow-up required
−Potential issues with willingness to be
randomized to interventions of interest
−Generalizability

META-ANALYSIS:RCTs
−Sample size needed for outcome
−Number, quality of RCTs
−Consistency of data reporting on variables
and outcome of interest
−Generalizability

**META-ANALYSIS: OBSERVATIONAL
STUDIES**
−Sample size needed for outcome
−Number, quality of relevant studies
−Consistency of data reporting on variables and
outcome of interest
−Duration of follow-up

OBSERVATIONAL STUDY:NEW DATA
−Sample size needed for outcome
−Size of pool of potential subjects
−Duration of follow-up
−Difficulty, cost of measurement

**OBSERVATIONAL STUDY: EXISTING
DATA**
−Sample size needed for outcome
−Availability of data
−Consistency of data reporting on variables
and outcome of interest

MODELING
−Availability of appropriate expertise
−Feasibility/cost/ethical issues of other study
designs

RCT? — Yes → RCT
No

Meta-analysis of RCTs? — Yes → Meta-analysis of RCTs
No

Meta-analysis: Observational — Yes → Meta-analysis of Observational Studies
No

Observational Study: New Data — Yes → New Data Collection
No

Observational Study: Existing Data — Yes → Analysis of Existing Data
No

Modeling — Yes → Modeling → Use Modeling Results to Reevaluate Feasiblity of Other Studies

We explore below in more detail the potential study designs represented in the Figure above and their specific considerations:

Randomized Controlled Trials (RCTs)

Ideally, all evidence gaps would be filled by conducting effectiveness RCTs that specifically address the area of interest; however, especially for many questions of interest for comparative effectiveness research, RCTs are rarely the most practical option. Considerations include:

- Sample size required for a particular outcome and to include a representative sample of patients: Many outcomes of interest, particularly those involving safety, are relatively uncommon, requiring an inordinately large sample size to achieve adequate power.
- Size of the pool of potential subjects: Some conditions may be relatively uncommon, or the subpopulation of interest relatively small, adversely affecting the sample size.
- Alternatively, comorbidities may be common among patients with the condition in question, creating potential difficulties with inclusion/exclusion criteria for an RCT.
- Duration of followup required: Minimizing loss to followup within the context of a trial, particularly if blinding must be maintained, is both expensive and difficult the longer the duration of followup, but for some outcomes lengthy followup is required.
- Issues with willingness to be randomized: Patient and provider beliefs about effectiveness, side effects, or other factors can make it difficult to recruit subjects into trials for some interventions.
- Generalizability: Inclusion/exclusion criteria often mean that subjects who participate in RCTs rarely reflect the full spectrum of either disease severity or co-morbidity that exists in the real world.

Meta-Analysis of RCTs

If a new RCT is not feasible, then a meta-analysis of existing RCTs may provide the next most valid answer to the question if studies are available; however, all of the potential difficulties with a new RCT are potential problems with existing RCTs. Given sufficient numbers and quality of existing RCTs, some questions may be addressable through meta-analysis. The main issue is whether data on the variables and outcomes of interest have been collected and reported consistently by enough RCTs to warrant a meta-analysis.

Meta-analysis of RCTs may be particularly appropriate for research gaps outside the scope of the initial CER; however, as highlighted by the authors of the original CER in their discussion of future research needs, this method may also be able answer key questions included in the original CER. Depending on the volume of ongoing research, existing reviews may quickly become out of date, particularly in cardiovascular research. In addition, when insufficient evidence exists for particular key questions, modifying the study inclusion/exclusion criteria from the initial review may allow broader inclusion of studies that can address these research gaps. This may be particularly true when a specific clinical condition, such as hypertension, has significant clinical overlap with related conditions such as ischemic heart disease, peripheral vascular disease, diabetes, chronic kidney disease, or congestive heart failure. When the outcomes of interest are common to all conditions (e.g., medication side effects, quality of life) then meta-analysis across clinical conditions may provide additional useful information. In meta-analyses of clinical trials, clinicians are often interested in examining subset effects, yet study-level analyses can lead to biased assessments and have some limitations in explaining heterogeneity. A meta-analysis of individual patient data offers several advantages for this purpose, but may not always be feasible given the multiple different sources of data and the proprietary nature of industry-sponsored research.

Meta-Analysis of Observational Studies

If a meta-analysis of RCTs is not feasible, the next most valid and feasible alternative would be a meta-analysis of observational studies. Many of the same issues inherent in meta-analyses of RCTs (both study-level and patient-level data) are also present, including:

- Heterogeneity in study design, inclusion, and exclusion criteria;
- Consistency in variable definitions and collection; and
- Varying duration of followup.

In addition, control of confounding can be especially challenging at the study level. Here, patient-level meta-analysis may be particularly appropriate, since it facilitates adjustment. The main challenge here is accessibility to the appropriate data, which may be difficult, especially with industry-sponsored studies.

Observational Study—Collection of New Data

If there is not sufficient literature available for a meta-analysis of observational data, then design of a new study would be the next most valid and feasible study design. Ideally, a prospective study with subject recruitment, data collection, and data analysis specifically intended to address the question of interest would be designed and carried out. Challenges to feasibility of a new observational study include:

- Duration of followup and retention: Many of the most important evidence gaps may require data on outcomes over a longer period of time. Subject retention is crucial both to maximize study power and minimize bias to differential dropout, but the resources required to maintain high retention over a long study period are substantial.
- Recruitment: Depending on the outcomes being assessed, participation in an ongoing observational study may be burdensome. Especially for patients treated with already approved treatments and whose clinical care is not affected by participation in a study, assuring maximal recruitment can be difficult. This may be a special problem in some populations with historically low levels of participation in research.

Observational Study—Analysis of Existing Data

If a new observational study is not feasible, there may be existing data available that address the relevant question. Major issues here include:

- Ease of access to data, particularly proprietary data from industry-sponsored trials or private health plans
- Extracting useful data from administrative or clinical records. ICD-9 (*International Classification of Diseases, Ninth Revision*) and CPT (*Current Procedural Terminology*) codes are not sensitive to many relevant factors in a patient's clinical history, or to disease severity within conditions. Paper records are difficult to abstract because of issues relating to legibility, consistency in diagnostic language, and the human resources required to convert clinical records into useful analytic data. Electronic medical records

are more useful, but are not universally used, and systems may not be compatible. For any of these sources, data on the variables of greatest interest may not have been consistently collected.

- Generalizability: Patients enrolled in Medicare, Medicaid, or private health plans may differ in a number of respects, such as income and employment history, that may be relevant, but which may be difficult to adjust for given the available data.

Modeling

Finally, if none of the above options is feasible, simulation modeling may be able to address some questions. Modeling is particularly helpful for addressing questions that involve very long durations of followup, or options that cannot feasibly be included in an RCT, such as the comparative impact of different screening frequencies on cancer incidence, mortality, and life expectancy. The main limitation here is the availability of appropriate expertise in both modeling and the clinical conditions being studied.

www.ingramcontent.com/pod-product-compliance
Lightning Source LLC
Chambersburg PA
CBHW081356170526
45166CB00010B/3110